Imprisoned Fathers

This volume specifically examines current concerns about imprisoned fathers and highlights best practices with a group of children and parents who present significant vulnerabilities. It brings together contemporary works in this area, to share and consolidate knowledge, to encourage comparisons and collaborations across jurisdictions, and to stimulate debate, all with the aim of furthering knowledge and improving practice in this area.

Although there is considerable focus on imprisoned mothers, there is limited knowledge or understanding of the needs, experiences, or effective responses to imprisoned fathers and their children, despite men making up the vast majority of the prison population. The ongoing and negative impact of parental incarceration on children is well documented, and includes emotional and behavioural consequences, marginalisation, and stigma, as well as financial and social stresses. However, understanding of these processes, and, importantly, what can assist children and families, is poor.

This book seeks to add to the understanding of paternal imprisonment by providing an in-depth exploration of how the arrest, detention, and experiences of fathers during imprisonment can affect their ability to parent and meet the needs of their children.

This book was originally published as a special issue of *Child Care in Practice*.

Catherine Flynn is a Senior Lecturer in the Department of Social Work at Monash University, Australia. Her core research area is the intersection of criminal justice and social work. She has a keen interest in understanding and addressing the wider and unintended consequences of criminal justice policy on families.

Michelle Butler is a Lecturer in Criminology at the School of Social Sciences, Education and Social Work at Queen's University Belfast, UK. Her core research areas include penology, parental imprisonment, penal reform, and criminological psychology.

Imprisoned Fathers

Responding to a Growing Concern

Edited by
Catherine Flynn and Michelle Butler

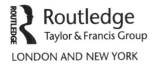
Routledge
Taylor & Francis Group

LONDON AND NEW YORK

First published 2019
by Routledge
2 Park Square, Milton Park, Abingdon, Oxon, OX14 4RN

and by Routledge
52 Vanderbilt Avenue, New York, NY 10017

First issued in paperback 2020

Routledge is an imprint of the Taylor & Francis Group, an informa business

British Library Cataloguing in Publication Data
A catalogue record for this book is available from the British Library

ISBN 13: 978-0-367-67133-4 (pbk)
ISBN 13: 978-0-367-19467-3 (hbk)

Typeset in Minion Pro
by RefineCatch Limited, Bungay, Suffolk

Publisher's Note
The publisher accepts responsibility for any inconsistencies that may have arisen
during the conversion of this book from journal articles to book chapters,
namely the possible inclusion of journal terminology.

Disclaimer
Every effort has been made to contact copyright holders for their permission to
reprint material in this book. The publishers would be grateful to hear from any
copyright holder who is not here acknowledged and will undertake to rectify
any errors or omissions in future editions of this book.

Contents

Citation Information

The chapters in this book were originally published in *Child Care in Practice*, volume 24, issue 2 (April 2018). When citing this material, please use the original page numbering for each article, as follows:

For any permission-related enquiries please visit:
http://www.tandfonline.com/page/help/permissions

Notes on Contributors

Tess S. Bartlett is a recent PhD graduate from the Department of Social Work, and a Teaching Associate in Criminology at Monash University, Australia. She researches the experiences of incarcerated primary carer fathers in Victoria, and masculinity.

Gwyneth Boswell is Director of Boswell Research Fellows, and Visiting Professor in the School of Health Sciences at the University of East Anglia, UK.

Katie Buston is a Senior Investigator Scientist at the MRC/CSO Social and Public Health Sciences Unit at the University of Glasgow, UK. She has been conducting research on fathers in prison for over ten years, as part of her broader research interest in children, young people, families, and health.

Michelle Butler is a Lecturer in Criminology at the School of Social Sciences, Education and Social Work at Queen's University Belfast, UK. Her core research areas include penology, parental imprisonment, penal reform, and criminological psychology.

John Devaney is Professor in Social Work at the University of Edinburgh, UK. He specialises in child abuse and neglect, family relationships, the impact of childhood adversity across the lifespan, and developing child welfare policy.

Fiona Donson is a Law Lecturer, and currently the Director of the Centre for Criminal Justice and Human Rights at University College Cork, Ireland. She researches and teaches in the areas of criminal justice, human rights, and administrative law.

Catherine Flynn is a Senior Lecturer in the Department of Social Work at Monash University, Australia. Her core research area is the intersection of criminal justice and social work. She has a keen interest in understanding and addressing the wider and unintended consequences of criminal justice policy on families.

Gunnar Vold Hansen is a Political Scientist and Professor at Østfold University College, Norway. His research topics have mainly focussed on integrated services for patients with concurrent addiction and mental health problems, and services for prisoners.

David Hayes is a Senior Lecturer in Social Work at Queen's University Belfast, UK. He specialises in childhood adversity, child wellbeing, child protection, and children's experiences of the criminal justice system.

Aisling Parkes is a Lecturer in Law at the Law School at University College Cork, Ireland. Her research areas include the rights of children affected by parental imprisonment, the rights of children in care, the right of the child to be heard, and children's rights in sport. She is co-Director of a sports law clinic for undergraduate law students.

Andrew Percy is a Senior Lecturer in Criminology at Queen's University Belfast, UK. He specialises in the alcohol and drug use of young people, research design and measurement, as well as evaluative research.

Melinda Tasca is an Assistant Professor in the Department of Criminal Justice and Criminology at Sam Houston State University, USA. Her research interests include correctional policy, the impact of incarceration on families, and the influence of race/ethnicity and gender in the criminal justice system.

Christopher J. Trotter is an Emeritus Professor in the Social Work Department at Monash University, Australia, and Director of the Monash Criminal Justice Research Consortium. Previously, he worked for many years as a community corrections officer and regional manager in the Victorian Department of Justice.

Imprisoned Fathers—Responding to Children

Many have commented on the invisibility of fathers in the area of child and family welfare in research, policy and practice (e.g. see Brown, Callahan, Strega, Walmsley, & Dominelli, 2009). This special edition of Child Care in Practice focuses on a much-overlooked issue in child and family scholarship: responding to the needs of children whose fathers are imprisoned.

In recent decades, we have seen growing recognition of the important role played by fathers in their children's lives and subsequently, the impact of absent fathers. It is now generally accepted that fathers have an important, and separate, role to play in children's lives and have a significant influence on how children grow and develop into adulthood (Fletcher, May, St George, Stoker, & Oshan, 2014; Huerta et al., 2013). Contemporary discourse encourages fathers to be "hands-on" in their parenting, promoting displays of men cuddling, playing with and feeding their children (Brown et al., 2009). Yet, there seems to be little guidance on how to achieve this state, particularly for those fathers who face challenges across a range of life domains, and perhaps need most help. There has also been a growing recognition that the term father should not just refer to those that are the biological fathers of children but should also include non-biological social and legal relationships, such as adoptive fathers, step-fathers, social fathers (i.e. where a man has assumed responsibility for a child), as well (see Marsiglio, Day, & Lamb, 2000).

The corollary of the present, active, good father, is the bad, absent father. Our understanding of what has become known as "father absence" is, in many ways, limited in focus. McLanahan, Tach, and Schneider (2013) provide evidence of the negative impact of father absence on children's school completion, social-emotional adjustment and their mental health as adults. However, this research only focused on father absence arising from parental divorce/ separation or father absence from birth. Less is known about father absence arising from imprisonment and the specific needs of imprisoned fathers and their children. McLanahan et al. (2013) also note that much research in this area has found it difficult to disentangle what causes the negative impacts of father absence from the circumstances that led to the father's absence and how these effects may intersect. If we consider parental incarceration as a very specific type of father absence, which typically co-occurs alongside other personal and structural issues, including substance abuse, mental health, family violence, poor education and employment, then it seems highly likely that these intersecting issues will create an even more negative impact on children.

Often, the impact of parental imprisonment on children is overshadowed in the minds of the general public and policymakers by the criminal status of the imprisoned father and focus on the father's offending behaviour. This is unfortunate as not only does it not consider how imprisonment can result in negative harms for innocent children but it also fails to appreciate how parental imprisonment may increase the risk of these children becoming involved in anti-social behaviour and crime in the future (Besemer, van der Geest, Murray, Bijleveld, & Farrington, 2011; Murray, Farrington, & Sekol, 2012). Greater attention needs to be paid to this area as we continue to imprison more people throughout the world, increasing the number of children that are affected by parental imprisonment.

Parental Imprisonment

In 2016, over 11 million people were believed to be imprisoned throughout the world, with the world prison population growing at a faster rate than the world's general population (20% compared to 18%) (Walmsley, 2016). While exact figures on the number of children affected by parental imprisonment are not available (as these statistics are not routinely collected by criminal justice authorities), estimates suggest that "probably tens of millions of children around the world" are affected by parental imprisonment (Robertson, 2012, p. 8). The vast majority of those imprisoned are men, with over 93% of those imprisoned globally identifying as male (Walmsley, 2016). Consequently, this special issue is focusing on the issues of imprisoned fathers as the vast majority of parents imprisoned are fathers.

It is important to note, however, that not all groups experience imprisonment equally. Some groups are more likely to be imprisoned than others, with minority groups and lower socio-economic groups being especially likely to be imprisoned (Tonry, 1997; Wacquant, 2009). Moreover, jurisdictions differ in their birth rate, with Africa and some parts of Asia and Oceania reporting above average global birth rates, while other areas such as Europe, North America, South America, Australia and New Zealand report below average global birth rates (United Nations, 2016). These figures suggest that some groups and some jurisdictions are more likely to be affected by parental imprisonment than others. In addition, large scale, quantitative studies have found that parental imprisonment can have significant long-term social, economic, behavioural and psychological consequences for children but that these effects can vary between different jurisdictions, depending on the availability of social supports, the wider political and economic context and the conditions of imprisonment in a particular jurisdiction (Besemer et al., 2011; Murray, Janson, & Farrington, 2007; Wilderman, 2014). The quality of father–child relationships prior to imprisonment and the extent to which family contact is maintained or restricted by criminal justice policies, practices and procedures can also influence the extent to which parental imprisonment can negatively impact on children (Dennison, Smallbone, & Occhipinti, 2017; Hutton, 2016; Sharrat, 2014).

This special issue seeks to add to our understanding of parental imprisonment by providing an in-depth exploration of how the arrest, detention and experiences of fathers during imprisonment can affect their ability to parent and meet the needs of their children. Contemporary scholarship from across the U.K., Ireland, Norway, the U.S.A. and Australia is drawn together to share and consolidate knowledge in this area, as well as stimulate debate, with the aim of furthering our understanding of how to effectively respond to the needs of imprisoned fathers and their children. This body of work also seeks to highlight the need for government policy and statutory welfare bodies to focus on the needs of children affected by parental imprisonment as a priority area and to recognise the importance of adopting a joined-up, coordinated response to this issue.

The special issue begins with Bartlett and colleagues highlighting how the needs of children in Australia are often forgotten about at the point of parental arrest and how greater attention needs to be paid to how such arrests are conducted to ensure that children are not traumatised or left without care. Next, Tasca discusses how the experience of incarceration in the U.S.A. may be transforming fatherhood and the role of fathers in the lives of their children. She examines how imprisonment can disrupt fathers' ability to parent but also describes how, for some, prison visiting may provide an opportunity to interrupt existing patterns and improve father–child relationships. Following on from this, Parkes and Donson examine how the experience of visiting prison in Ireland has usually not been structured in such a way that considers the rights of children or their needs. They argue that prison visitation needs to respect children's rights and consider the impact of visitation on children. In attempting to maintain family relationships, prison based parenting programmes can often be used. The next three papers focus on programmes supporting fathers in three different jurisdictions. In Scotland, Buston and colleagues discuss the challenges that can be encountered in attempting to recruit, retain and engage young fathers in such a programme. Hayes and colleagues build on this to highlight the importance of a programme in Northern Ireland that is providing opportunities for fathers to rehearse the new skills they are acquiring, so they can master these skills and use them to improve father–child relationships and meet the needs of their children. Similarly, Hansen examines such a programme in Norway, demonstrating how it can help improve fathers' parenting skills and father–child contact. He concludes, however, that such programmes are limited in their ability to help families with the wider economic and social challenges they face, unless there is a more comprehensive and coordinated approach to the needs of these children and families across the social welfare and criminal justice systems. Then, Boswell offers some personal reflections on why a more comprehensive and coordinated approach to the needs of children with imprisoned fathers has not been adopted in England and Wales. She points to a number of weaknesses in existing research (many of which can be seen in the studies included in this special issue), as well as a lack of official statistics and the politicisation of crime as contributing to the failure to adopt a coordinated, joined-up approach to this issue.

This special edition, therefore, seeks to draw attention to the needs of children with imprisoned fathers, and to contribute to consolidating knowledge, stimulating debate and focusing attention on addressing gaps and weaknesses in our knowledge. This will enable pressure to be increased on policymakers, politicians and statutory bodies to prioritise this issue and adopt a more coordinated, joined-up approach to addressing the needs of these children.

References

Besemer, S., van der Geest, V., Murray, J., Bijleveld, C. C. J. H., & Farrington, D. P. (2011). The relationship between parental imprisonment and offspring offending in England and the Netherlands. *British Journal of Criminology, 51*(2), 413–437.

Brown, L., Callahan, M., Strega, S., Walmsley, C., & Dominelli, L. (2009). Manufacturing ghost fathers: The paradox of father presence and absence in child welfare. *Child and Family Social Work, 14*, 25–34.

Davies A. (2009, June 23). Be there, says Obama, a son whose dad wasn't. *The Age,* 8.

Dennison, S., Smallbone, H., & Occhipinti, S. (2017). Understanding how incarceration challenges proximal processes in father-child relationships: Perspectives of imprisoned fathers. *Journal of Developmental and Life-Course Criminology 3*(1), 15–38.

Fletcher, R., May, C., St George, J., Stoker, L., & Oshan, M. (2014). *Engaging fathers: Evidence review.* Canberra: Australian Research Alliance for Children and Youth.

Huerta, M. C., Adema, W., Baxter, J., Han, W. J., Lausten, M., Lee, R., & Waldfogel, J. (2013). *Fathers' leave, fathers' involvement and child development: Are they related? Evidence from four OECD countries.* No 140, OECD social, employment and migration working papers. Paris: OECD Publishing.

Hutton, M. (2016). Visiting time. *Probation Journal, 63*(3), 347–361.

Marsiglio, W., Day, R. D., & Lamb, M. E. (2000). Exploring fatherhood diversity: Implications for conceptualizing father involvement. *Marriage & Family Review, 29*(4), 269–293.

McLanahan, S., Tach, L., & Schneider, D. (2013). The causal effects of father absence. *Annual Review of Sociology, 39*, 399–427.

Murray, J., Farrington, D. P., & Sekol, I. (2012). Children's antisocial behavior, mental health, drug use, and educational performance after parental incarceration: A systematic review and meta-analysis. *Psychological Bulletin, 138*(2), 175–210.

Murray, J., Janson, C.-G., & Farrington, D. P. (2007). Crime in adult offspring of prisoners – A cross-national comparison of two longitudinal samples. *Criminal Justice and Behavior, 34*(1), 133–149.

Robertson, O. (2012). *Collateral convicts: Children of incarcerated parents.* Geneva: The Quaker United Nations Office.

Sharrat, K. (2014). Children's experiences of contact with imprisoned parents: A comparison between four European countries. *European Journal of Criminology, 11*(6), 760–775.

Tonry, M. (1997). Ethnicity, crime and immigration. *Crime and Justice: A Review of Research, 21,* 1–29.

United Nations. (2016). *World fertility patterns 2015.* Geneva: United Nations.

Wacquant, L. (2009). *Punishing the poor: The neoliberal government of social insecurity.* London: Duke University Press.

Walmsley, R. (2016). *World prison population list* (11th ed.). London: Institute for Criminal Policy Research.

Wilderman, C. (2014). Parental incarceration, child homelessness, and the invisible consequences of mass imprisonment. *The ANNALS of the American Academy of Political and Social Science, 651*(1), 74–96.

Catherine Flynn

Michelle Butler

"They Didn't Even Let Me Say Goodbye": A Study of Imprisoned Primary Carer Fathers' Care Planning for Children at the Point of Arrest in Victoria, Australia

Tess S. Bartlett ⓘ, Catherine A. Flynn ⓘ and Christopher J. Trotter ⓘ

ABSTRACT

In Victoria, data indicates that in 2013–2014 there were 74,992 adult male arrests, yet little formal attention has been paid to the parenting status of these men, despite knowledge of the impact of parental arrest and incarceration on children being well established. This article addresses a gap in the literature by providing new insights into the experiences of arrest of 34 primary carer fathers incarcerated in Victoria. It examines how incarcerated primary carer fathers experience planning processes for their children at the time of arrest and what factors facilitate or hinder the planning process. To do so, the article draws on data gathered for an Australian Research Council funded study conducted in Victoria and New South Wales between 2011 and 2015. Key issues include: the primary location of paternal arrest; the presence, or absence, of children at the location at which the arrest is made; police awareness of children; and subsequent discussions between police and fathers about suitable care. Findings indicate that half of all arrests took place in the family home. Children were present in 10 of these arrests and half were characterised by force, a large number of police, or weapons. Findings also indicate that in around one-half of all arrests, children were not physically present, despite fathers continuing to have responsibilities for these children. Despite 27 of the arrested men reporting that the police were aware (or made aware) of their children, almost all of these men ($n = 26$) were not asked about suitable care even when their children were physically present. Overall qualitative findings depict an absence of any discussion about children between police and fathers during the arrest process. The study highlights the demand for guidelines regarding child sensitive practice when a primary carer father is arrested.

Introduction

The current article examines imprisoned primary carer fathers' accounts of their arrest[1] process, with a specific focus on factors which affected how they were able to fulfil their responsibilities to their dependent children. Due to the lack of existing research relating to imprisoned primary carer fathers and arrest, the paper begins with a discussion of research examining parental, and where possible paternal, imprisonment before moving on to parental arrest, to understand the specific needs of this group; limitations are noted appropriately. Research findings and implications are presented, drawn from one aspect of an Australian Research Council (ARC) study, "The Impact of Incarceration on Children's Care: A Strategic Framework for Good Care Planning, 2011–2014", which examined responses to children when their primary carer was arrested and imprisoned in Victoria and New South Wales (for details see Trotter et al., 2015).

Review of literature

Parental incarceration and children

There has been considerable growth noted in prison populations globally (Walmsley, 2016). Subsequent research has investigated and described the impact of parental incarceration on children (see, for example, Brown, Dibb, Shenton, & Elson, 2001; Dennison & Smallbone, 2015; Johnston & Gabel, 1995; Nurse, 2002; Wright & Seymour, 2000).

Given that the vast majority of prisoners are men (e.g. see ABS, 2016; Glaze & Kaeble, 2014), with international evidence indicating that around 50% of these men are parents (Glaze & Maruschak, 2008), recent years have seen some research drawing specific attention to fathers in prison. Studies have examined: situated fathering and the visit space in the United Kingdom (UK) (Moran, 2017); fathering identity in prisons in Hong Kong and in England (Chui, 2016; Meek, 2011); challenges and barriers facing incarcerated Indigenous fathers (Dennison, Smallbone, Stewart, Freiberg, & Teague, 2014) and parental involvement for incarcerated fathers in Queensland (Dennison & Smallbone, 2015); and the intergenerational transmission of offending between fathers and children in South Australia (Halsey & Deegan, 2012).

In Australia, the exact number of children affected by paternal imprisonment remains unknown. An Australian Institute of Health and Welfare (AIHW) study noted in 2015 that 46% of the 1011 male "prison entrants"[2] had at least one dependent child prior to imprisonment (AIHW, 2015, p. 8). Yet only 49% of prison entrants overall (both men and women combined) took part in the study. United States (US) data (The Pew Charitable Trusts, 2010) indicates there are an estimated 2.7 million dependent children affected by paternal imprisonment, a figure that increased by 77% between 1991 and 2004 (Glaze & Maruschak, 2008). In the Australian context there is limited data, but Queensland research estimates that in any given year some 0.8% of children in that state will be affected by paternal incarceration and 4% in their lifetime (Dennison, Stewart, & Freiberg, 2013).

It is clear then that while existing research provides some insight into parental incarceration more generally, there remains a considerable gap in knowledge regarding fathers in direct caring roles, with paternal arrest preceding imprisonment a potentially traumatising time for children.

Parental arrest

Research examining the processes of and responses to parental arrest is limited. One study, conducted in California, sought to specifically investigate the responses of law enforcement agencies, as well as child welfare organisations, at the point of arrest (Nieto,

2002). Findings indicate that the period following arrest was a time of uncertainty for children with limited communication between families and agencies involved (Nieto, 2002). The effects of children's exposure to a traumatic event, such as an arrest, have also been noted by The Yale Child Study Center (2011) and include *inter alia*: loss of sleep, separation anxiety, hyper-vigilance, irritability, and withdrawal. Another study in the US examined child exposure to parental criminal activity, arrest, and sentencing, and the relationship to child maladjustment (Dallaire & Wilson, 2010). The study found that witnessing parental arrest might be detrimental to children and raised the risk of problem behaviours. Another US study that sought to examine the relationship between witnessing an arrest and elevated post-traumatic stress disorder (PTSD) (American Psychiatric Association, 2016) symptoms indicated that witnessing a parent's arrest can be particularly traumatic even when other PTSD explanations are taken into account (Phillips & Zhao, 2010). Further, that witnessing an arrest "is a distinct predictor of children's elevated PTS[D] symptoms" (Phillips & Zhao, 2010, p. 1253).

Data also tends to focus predominantly on mothers (see Annie E. Casey Foundation [AECF], 2001; Lilburn, 2001; Nieto, 2002) or relate to the impact of multiple/traumatic events on children, for instance, arrest *and* imprisonment (see Dallaire & Wilson, 2010; Simmons, 2000; The Yale Child Study Center, 2011). Nieto's (2002) research provides a clear example of the use of gender neutral terms, as it is about mothers, yet is labelled as being about "parents" thus obscuring understanding of the, perhaps, differing experiences for mothers and fathers. Such research does, however, highlight the harmful effects of parental arrest on children, and shows that these events continue to be characterised by disordered and ad hoc practices. Concurrently, data collection about parenting/dependent children is also limited and arguably ad hoc. In Victoria, although data is collected regarding the location of offences (Victoria Police, 2013), the primary carer status of offenders at the point of arrest is not routinely collected. The only related data available on this shows that during 2013–2014 there were 74,992 adult male arrests (Victoria Police, 2014). Based on data above that indicates 46% of male prison entrants had at least one dependent child prior to imprisonment (AIHW, 2015), we estimate that around 30,000 of these are likely to be parents, although any further detail about parenting or caring status is unknown.

Formal responses to children at parental arrest

The chaotic nature of arrest procedures was highlighted by caregivers from Dallaire and Wilson's (2010) research and highlights the need for formal responses. Nieto (2002) also found clear gaps in formal responses to children. Less than half (42%) of law enforcement officers stated that they would enquire about the care of child/ren present at the arrest of their parent/s; when children were not physically present, only 13% of respondents advised they would make enquiries. A subsequent smaller survey of 38 police officers in Michigan indicated similar findings, with responses indicating a distinct lack of communication and policy regarding children at the point of arrest (Neville, 2010). Earlier research by Lilburn (2001) examining police arrest practices for women and their dependent children in South Australia resulted in similar findings. Police acknowledged that children's care arrangements needed to be made when a mother was taken into custody, yet it was not considered a significant problem. Furthermore, police tended to rely on "common sense" at the point of arrest to make contact with partners, friends, other family members, or welfare services, with an assumption that care was available for these children (Lilburn, 2001). Existing research thus highlights the competing obligations for police when on duty: the obligation to follow police procedures as well as their duty of care to children.

When reflecting on formal responses that have been implemented outside Australia, one can see evidence of several child sensitive arrest procedures in US jurisdictions. Alongside the co-location and/or joint training of child welfare and law enforcement officers in California (Puddefoot & Foster, 2007), the US International Association of Chiefs of Police (IACP), with funding support from the Department of Justice (DOJ), recently developed a Model Policy aimed to "address the needs of children at the time of, and just following, their parent's arrest" (IACP, 2014, p. ix). In particular, the policy seeks to assist law enforcement agencies and partner organisations in developing measures to safeguard children when a parent is arrested. The policy statement notes that officers will be "trained to identify and respond effectively to a child, present or not present, whose parent is arrested" to help minimise trauma and promote child safety following arrest (IACP, 2014, p. 8). This policy refers specifically to children of arrested parents, whilst also acknowledging children who are not present at the time of the arrest. The IACP also currently offer no-cost training, technical assistance and resources for law enforcement to mitigate trauma experienced by children who have parents in the criminal justice system (IACP, 2016). Other child appropriate responses have been initiated in Sweden, where offenders take part in an interview at the police station that involves questions about care arrangements for children (Mulready-Jones, 2011). Where there are no long-term arrangements for children, there is a duty on the police to inform Children's Services.

In Victoria there has been very little advancement of this sort. The Department of Health and Human Services (DHHS[3])—Child Protection—is responsible for the protection of children under the Children, Youth and Families Act, 2005 (Vic). Under the 2005 Act, police have statutory responsibilities and are classified as protective interveners and have a legal mandate to intervene when a child is in need of protection. The *Victoria Police Manual-Guidelines* (Victoria Police, 2017) require supervisors to enquire if a person at arrest is a primary carer and if so to enquire if suitable arrangements have been made to care for that child. Police responsibilities are also outlined in the *Protecting Children: Protocol between Department of Health and Human Services, Child Protection and Victoria Police* (DHHS, 2012; herein referred to as the *DHHS Protocol*). The *DHHS Protocol* establishes how the two services work together to meet their respective legislative mandates and to achieve positive outcomes in the best interests of the child/ren. It advises that officers, in their role of protective interveners, *must consider* making a report to Child Protection where it is believed a child is in need of protection in situations including abandonment or parental incapacitation. It is noted that this:

> … may include situations where a primary carer of dependent children is in custody and incapable of caring for their child during this period and there is no other suitable person willing or able to care for the child. (DHHS, 2012, p. 11)

Importantly, both the *Victoria Police Manual* and the *DHHS Protocol* do not provide any further guidance as to assessing parental incapacitation or carer suitability, with these terms open to considerable interpretation. Flynn, Naylor, and Fernandez (2015) note that officers who are aware of children consider it to be part of their duty of care to make enquiries and ensure their safety, particularly when children are physically present at arrest. Yet these actions seem driven by a sense of individual responsibility, rather than a formal process. Flynn, Bartlett, Fernandez Arias, Evans, and Burgess (2015) also found that gathering of informal knowledge was more likely to occur in rural, rather than metropolitan, areas. Child sensitive responses, however, are highly influenced by the physical presence of children, with one police participant stating "We naturally assume that if they don't have custody of the children at the time [at arrest] then it's, then there's no issue" (Flynn, Naylor, et al., 2015, p. 10). While some jurisdictions are implementing innovative practices, it remains clear that fathers as carers, along with their children, are largely overlooked at the point of arrest. While it is known, generally, that parental incarceration has a negative impact on children, an understanding of the specific implications of paternal incarceration, and more specifically arrest, is absent.

Methodology

Using incarcerated primary carer fathers' experiences of arrest, this article addresses the following research question:

> How do primary carer fathers experience planning processes for their children at the time of arrest and what factors facilitate or hinder the planning process?

The study aims to address a gap in research by providing new insights into the experiences of incarcerated primary carer fathers at the point of arrest. For the purposes of this article, primary carer status is defined by three outcome-focused criteria: their child/ren required a new carer (relative, friend, or associate) to take over their care in their own home; their child/ren were required to move to a new house to live with a different carer; or their child/ren were left with no carer.

Recruitment

Data was collected from imprisoned primary carer fathers from May 2012 to October 2013. Stratified purposive sampling (Patton, 2002) was used to select a representation of maximum, medium, and minimum security settings from prisons in Victoria and NSW. Prisons were identified in conjunction with the relevant correctional service departments as suitable data collection sites, on the basis of security rating and numbers of known parents. Two correctional settings were purposefully excluded at this point in the process due to the nature of the offences committed by a number of prisoners (specifically child sex offences), which prevented follow up with families, and three of the settings declined due to lack of capacity/operational reasons. Data was ultimately gathered from three settings ($n = 9$, $n = 14$, and $n = 16$), covering all security classifications.

Once entry was approved, a variety of recruitment methods were used to locate participants, namely flyer display and distribution and communication with prison contact people (including programme officers and coordinators, clinical and integration services managers, social workers, project managers and prison officers). This yielded 23 participants; further targeting was employed by way of group sessions with prisoner peer educators to generate further discussion and pass on information to other prisoners. Participants took part in the study if they volunteered to participate, and were available at the time of the interview and thus received non-monetary compensation (for time out of cell and/or work) for taking part.

Data collection

This study used a multi-method approach to data collection, where the use of structured interviews sought both qualitative and quantitative data. This approach is particularly useful when examining new areas of study and sensitive areas of research (Liamputtong, 2007). It maximises the study's capacity to capture a holistic view of issues experienced by fathers, as well as allowing for clear cross-case analysis. Interviews were conducted face-to-face and focused on key decision-making and transition points. Due to security constraints within the prison setting, audio recording was not permitted. Comprehensive note taking was instead employed to document the data. Once the interviews were complete, qualitative data was analysed using content analysis via NVivo10. Ethical oversight of the project involved a total of nine Human Research Ethics Committees (HREC) or Research Coordinating Committees (RCC) reviewing and approving the project.[4]

Sample

For the purposes of this paper, data from the 34 imprisoned primary carer fathers arrested in Victoria is examined. All participants had been in prison for at least three months. The demographics of the sample group and their children are shown in Tables 1 and 2 below.

This specific sample shows some general similarities with the broader male prison population, with regard to average age and number of children, but also some differences, notably cultural groupings (ABS, 2016). These were not examined further in the study.

Interviews

Participants for this study were asked three questions by the lead author relating specifically to arrest, including (1) the circumstances of the arrest (and whether their children were present or not); (2) whether they believed the police officer was aware they were the primary carer of children; and (3) whether a discussion about suitable care took place. Data is presented below in response to these three areas.

Results

Initial analysis revealed differences in how men were able to engage in planning for their children, according to the location of arrest, such as whether it was in the home or in the

Table 1. Key characteristics of primary carer father participants.

Mean age (years)	Age range (years)	Australian born	Indigenous	Participants who report previous imprisonments	Total number of children	Age range of children (years)	Participants' care of children pre-prison	
							Full time	Shared care
39	25–52	28 (82%)	6 (18%)	24 (71%)	86	0–17	68 (79%)	18 (21%)

Table 2. Key characteristics of the children of primary carer father participants.

			Participants' care of children pre-prison	
Total number of children	Mean age (years)	Age range of children (years)	Full time	Shared care
86	9	0–17	68 (79%)	18 (21%)

community, whether participants reported there was use of force at the time of the arrest (including multiple police officers, Special Operations Group (SOG), weapons, raids or threats), as well as the likelihood of children being present and subsequent responses to this. Data has therefore been analysed accordingly.

Presence of children at time of arrest

Thirty-three respondents provided data about the circumstances of their arrest (the other respondent did not provide information regarding location of arrest). Figures 1 and 2 show a breakdown of data relating to arrests in the home and in the community respectively.

As indicated in Figures 1 and 2, children were present at almost a third of all arrests ($n = 11$) with data showing clear patterns relating to the location of the arrest. As seen in Figure 1, nearly half of the arrests ($n = 16$) took place in the home and children were present at 10 of these arrests. Participants described these processes and circumstances as follows:

> [I was at] home, children just gone to the shop. Knocked on the door …. They've known me for twenty years so they're pretty pleasant, they don't handcuff me in front of the kids or any-thing if they know they're there. (Craig)[5]

> [I was] at home and children were present when the police came. (Jack)

> [I was] at home getting ready to leave at 5.30am and police turned up and arrested me. (Leighton)

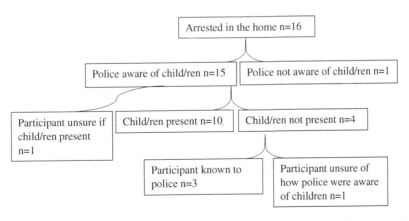

Figure 1. Primary carer fathers arrested in the home and police awareness of dependent child/ren.

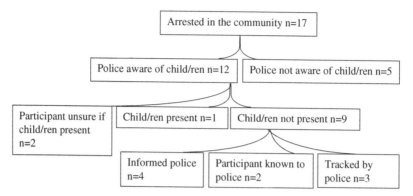

Figure 2. Primary carer fathers arrested in the community and police awareness of dependent child/ren.

As can be seen in Figure 2, in the community, there is a stark contrast, where children were largely absent ($n = 9/17$). This indicates, unsurprisingly, that when arresting a primary carer in the family home, it is likely that children will be present.

As is shown in Figure 2, 17 arrests took place in the community and, as described above, children were absent in nine of these cases: they were reported to be with either another parent or a family member, at school, or their presence was unknown or unidentified:

> I was in the back street of factories and the SOG's grabbed me and my partner. My kids were with my mum. (Alex)

> [The arrest] was in the community in [suburb], children were at school at the time. (Bob)

> Children weren't present. In [suburb], the C.I.U [Crime Investigation Unit] had me on surveillance. Two weeks prior I was arrested and charged with two burgs. Jumped out guns blazing and arrested me, so I'm glad the kids weren't there with ten guns pointed at me. (Craig)

> [I was] in [the] city, left kids at home, saw my mates, one thing led to another and it was armed robbery charge. (Nick)

Data illustrates that when arrests are made in the community children are less likely to be physically present. As will be discussed below, the presence of children is described by fathers as having some impact on police awareness of these children and some impact on response.

Police awareness

Participants were asked for their views on whether the police were aware of their primary carer role. Figures 1 and 2 above present data relating to this. In around 80% of cases (27: $n = 15$ arrested in the home and $n = 12$ in the community), participants noted that police were aware of their primary carer status. For those arrested in the family home, all but one participant reported that police were aware of their children due, in large part, to the physical presence of at least one child.

> Yes, I'd had three raids beforehand, so they were aware of it. (Vin)

Yes, they just saw the children. (Garry)

As seen in Figure 2 for those arrests that took place in the community, police were reported to be aware of the participant's primary carer status in the majority of cases ($n = 12$). Interestingly, this was typically *not* due to the presence of children, but rather because either the participant informed the police of their children ($n = 4$), the participant was known to or had a history with the police ($n = 2$), or they were under surveillance by the police ($n = 3$).

> Yes, I told them and they wouldn't give me bail because I wouldn't give them information. Kids were at their mother's at the time. Makes no difference to police if your kids are sitting at home alone or what. (Lou)

> Yes, had been arrested by them before for previous offence, but they didn't mention children [this time]. (Craig)

> Yes I think that's what they put out over the radio because they said I kidnapped my partner and child, so they knew. (Alex)

> Yes, I was under investigation for a while. (Don)

As data indicates, in over three-quarters of arrests, both in the home and in the community, fathers report that the police were aware of their primary carer status regardless of whether children are present or not. What can be deduced, therefore, is that police in this sample are typically aware of the primary carer status of offenders; however, this does not necessarily equate to having an understanding of men's primary caring role as indicated by the discussion below.

Discussions about suitable care

Participants were asked whether a discussion about suitable care for their dependent children took place at the point of arrest, initiated either by the arresting officer or by the participant. While the majority of participants indicate that police were aware of their dependent children, Figures 1 and 2 reveal that almost all of these men ($n = 26$) report that no subsequent discussion ensued regarding suitable care for their children. As Table 3 shows, this was the case irrespective of children's presence/absence during the arrest.

For those 26 participants who reported that no discussion about suitable care took place with the arresting officer, arrest locations were quite evenly spread between the community ($n = 12$) and in the home ($n = 13$) (one participant did not state whether his children were present or not). In only eight cases did discussions about suitable care take place and

Table 3. Incarcerated primary carer fathers' reports of discussions with arresting police officers about children's care arrangements and children's presence.

	Discussion	No discussion	Total
Child present	3	8	11
Child not present	5	14	19
Child's presence unknown	0	4	4
Total	8	26	34

this occurred where the police were aware of the participant's primary carer status, although this was not necessarily due to the child's *physical* presence.

Even in the 11 cases where the child/ren were present (*n* = 10 home, *n* = 1 community), only three participants recalled being asked/having discussions about suitable care and if there was a family member to call.

> Yes. Asked where was my daughter at the time. I let them know she was with her grand-mother. (Lewis)

> Yes, they asked if I had people that could look after them and care for them (children). Police officer that arrested me asked. (Pete)

> Yes, asked me if there was anyone to look after them or they would find care. (Lance)

For the remaining eight arrests, no discussion about suitable care took place. These were planned arrests in the home and were characterised by force, multiple police officers, weapons, raids, or were threatening.

> The children were present. [I] started punching people in the face because they had guns in my face. Guns in two year old daughter's face. It really affected them, seeing guns in Dad's face. (Bruce)

> All my kids were present, they came in very hard because it was an armed robbery ... and had the Special Operations Group (SOG). My kids were terrified ... My 12 year old now hates the police, which is bad because I never wanted him to do that. (Grant)

> It was unexpected. It was 6.30am – 7.00am. The coppas [*sic*] came and bashed on the door – about 30 of them. Oldest daughter opened the front door, they came barging in and arrested me. (David)

This suggests that, currently, when arresting an adult for a serious offence in the home, where children are likely to be present, the focus is *only* on the arrest, despite knowledge, or presence, of children.

In the 19 arrests where child/ren were not present (*n* = 4 home, *n* = 15 community), only five fathers engaged with arresting officers in a discussion about suitable care. In these cases, police had been tracking the individual prior to the arrest or the offender was known to the police. In three of these cases it was the participant who informed officers about their children, rather than a question being asked as part of police procedure.

> Yes, told them to ring me Mrs and to look after the kids until I got bail. So they rang her. (Nick)

> Yes, I told 'em. (Pete)

It is clear that when children are not present, discussions involving suitable care are unlikely to take place.

Discussion

Using incarcerated primary carer fathers' accounts of arrest, the current article aimed to respond to the research question "How do primary carer fathers experience planning processes for their children at the time of arrest and what factors facilitate or hinder the planning process?" This was done by identifying: the circumstances of paternal arrest—ascertaining the presence, or absence, of children; determining whether police were aware of a father's primary carer status; and finally exploring what, if any, discussions about suitable care for children took place. In doing so the article examined the extent to which fathers' caring responsibilities are taken into consideration during the arresting process, as determined by the circumstances of their arrest. This paper acknowledges there are a number of limitations to the study. Notably, the absence of children's views on the role of primary carer fathers in their lives limits the capacity to completely capture notions of paternal primary care and the direct experience for children. As well as this, the accounts analysed in this study are from imprisoned fathers only and there is an absence of police views regarding the behaviour, or experiences, of arresting officers with those specific cases. A further limitation is that while not all men were arrested in crisis mode, there may have been factors that influenced their perceptions of arresting procedures. Prisoner intoxication or substance status was not asked about. For some participants the interviews took place months after their arrest[6] and there is always the possibility of memory distortion. Consequently, this study is reliant on incarcerated fathers' recall of arrest and results must be viewed as such.

Nearly half of all arrests took place in the family home. Children were present in 10 of these, and half were characterised by force, a large number of police, or weapons. Making arrests in the family home could therefore act as a caution for police that children are likely to be present. The finding that children are more likely to be present in the family home corresponds with data from Dallaire and Wilson (2010), which indicates that children living with their parent prior to arrest are more likely to experience an arrest. While primary carer status was not determined in their study, it adds to our argument that, for law enforcement, arresting a parent in the home is likely to involve the presence of children. No research is currently available on the location of (parental) arrests in Victoria, although data is collected regarding the location of the offence (see Victoria Police, 2013). This signifies its level of prioritisation when, in reality, knowing more about arrest location would allow for better planning of such events and, ultimately, better responses to children.

In around one-half of arrests, children were not physically present despite fathers continuing to have responsibilities for these children. While absent children do not require physical attention during the arrest process, their needs still require consideration in order to diminish the potential impact on these children. This supports findings from Victoria based on data from police officers (Flynn, Naylor, et al., 2015), which established that when children are not physically present, the likelihood of them being considered is minimal. As mentioned previously, the *DHHS Protocol* suggests the need for consideration of primary carer responsibilities at the time of arrest (DHHS, 2012). Our research suggests that this should include the consideration of children, whether they are physically present at arrest, or not. Further, that child sensitive practices are required *regardless* of the arrest location.

A better response would be a planned response, similar to that implemented in Sweden (Mulready-Jones, 2011), with child sensitive procedures, interviews, and care arrangements made regardless of location. It is understood that for serious offences, safety is paramount and arrest protocols must be adhered to. However, child sensitive processes are more than simply procedures for responding well to children who are present at arrest.

At present, while there are some good, albeit ad hoc, child-aware practices in Victoria for police officers, as outlined in Flynn, Naylor, et al. (2015), despite this, there are poor, and poorly understood, guidelines in place for dealing with children when arresting a primary carer. Based on past research with arrested mothers (Lilburn, 2001), a child sensitive approach would involve giving fathers the opportunity to respond to, and deal with, their children at arrest. This would give fathers the ability to then take part in the planning process for their children. Furthermore, limiting forceful arrests that take place in the presence of children could potentially reduce short-term, and long-term, "risks" for children by reducing the likelihood of trauma that is known to take place when witnessing parental arrest (Dallaire & Wilson, 2010). Flynn, Bartlett, et al. (2015) note that police participants in their study reported greater levels of informal knowledge relating to offenders' families and children in rural/regional areas. Future research might investigate further whether this knowledge then impacts on the level of discussion that takes place between arresting officers and offenders about suitable care. Currently, there is limited discussion regarding care and even less if the children are not present. "Seeing" children is not enough. Instead, practices could involve protocols similar to those implemented in the US that provide training and resources for dealing with children in traumatic situations (IACP, 2014; Nieto, 2002). In particular, it is moving beyond education towards collaborative practice, such as the Model Policy initiated between child welfare and law enforcement officers in California. Such a policy would assist law enforcement and key child welfare services in developing measures to safeguard children when their parent is arrested.

Despite 27 of the arrested men (around 80%) reporting the police were aware (or made aware) of their children, almost all of these men ($n=26$) were not asked about suitable care even when their children were physically present. This may indicate gendered views held by police regarding primary care, with a subsequent assumption that men had a female partner somewhere to care for the child/ren. This was not specifically examined, however, in this study. It is worth considering the extent to which this finding is also affected by police understandings of their role with regard to children and responding to them at the point of arrest. Future research might explore the extent to which police assumptions regarding gender roles instigate practice, as differing masculine ideas may prompt different responses. While this article focuses specifically on fathers, it raises the question as to whether arrests of primary carer mothers would have been dealt with in the same manner.[7] It is not enough to simply encourage discussions about suitable care. Responding to children at the point of arrest would thus involve "seeing" men as fathers, and in turn challenge existing ideas that exist regarding the role of the father in society. Rather than discussions being about "mothers" versus "fathers" in the criminal justice system, the focus could instead be on primary carers and centred on children. This would mean a system based on the needs of all involved, rather than a select few.

At present, the lack of attention given to incarcerated primary carer fathers at the point of arrest is demonstrated by the limited formal response mechanisms that exist. The *DHHS Protocol* (DHHS, 2012) includes some direction to police officers for responding to children when parents are "incapacitated" and there is no other suitable person willing and available to care for the child. While it would be reasonably expected that police, in their role as protective interveners, would consider an arrested parent to be "incapacitated" and incapable of caring for his children, the protocol does not outline specific guidance regarding parental arrest. Overall, then, in Victoria, there is currently no policy or guidance around specific child sensitive arrest procedures as are being developed in other jurisdictions. This is despite the growing body of research indicating that witnessing parental arrest can be traumatising for children in both the short, and long, term (Phillips & Zhao, 2010). While based on a small and specific sample, this paper highlights the demand for such guidelines for this often overlooked group, with evidence depicting arrest procedures where there is an absence of any routine questioning around children. Even when the existence of children is known, discussions around suitable care are reported to be sparse. The challenge, then, is to consider the caring responsibilities for primary carer fathers at the point of arrest and thus prioritise children.

Notes

1. For the purposes of this article, arrest is defined according to the Crimes Act (Victoria) 1958.
2. A prison entrant was defined as a person 18 years or over entering full-time custody on remand or on a sentence (AIHW, 2015).
3. Previously the Department of Human Services (DHS).
4. These consisted of Monash University HREC, Victorian Department of Justice and its NSW counterpart Corrective Services, Department of Human Services Victoria and Family and Community Services in NSW, police in both states, and the Department of Education and Early Childhood Development in Victoria, as well as the Department of Education and Communities in NSW.
5. All names and places have been changed to respect the confidentiality of participants.
6. As this study was drawn from a larger ARC linkage project (Trotter et al., 2015) that focused on the impact of *incarceration* on children's care questions asked of participants were focused on care planning for children at the point of arrest, sentencing and imprisonment and time since arrest was not included.
7. Trotter et al. (2015) found that across Victoria and New South Wales there was indeed a gendered response across all arrest data for mothers and fathers, where women were significantly more likely to be asked about suitable care by an arresting officer or station sergeant than men.

Acknowledgements

This study was conducted with the support of key partner organisations: Department of Justice and Regulation (DOJR), Victoria, Department of Health and Human Services (DHHS) Victoria, Commission for Children and Young People (CCYP), Victorian Association for the Care and Resettlement of Offenders (VACRO), Prison Fellowship (PF) and SHINE for Kids (SHINE). Feedback on earlier drafts of this paper was gratefully received from Victoria Police.

Disclosure statement

No potential conflict of interest was reported by the authors.

Funding

This work was supported by the [Australian Research Council] under Grant [number LP110100084].

ORCID

Tess S. Bartlett ⓘ http://orcid.org/0000-0002-7211-757X
Catherine A. Flynn ⓘ http://orcid.org/0000-0001-7645-3469
Christopher J. Trotter ⓘ http://orcid.org/0000-0003-1812-9550

References

ABS. (2016). *Prisoners in Australia*, 2016 (No. 4517.0). Retrieved from http://www.abs.gov.au/ausstats/abs@.nsf/mf/4517.0

AIHW. (2015). *The health of Australia's prisoners* 2015 (Cat. no. PHE 170). Canberra: Author.

American Psychiatric Association. (2016). Post-traumatic Stress Disorder. Retrieved from http://www.apa.org/topics/ptsd/

Annie E.Casey Foundation (2001). Partnerships between Corrections and Child Welfare. US: The Women s Prison Association & Home, Inc.

Australian Bureau of Statistics, see ABS

Australian Institute of Health and Welfare, see AIHW

Brown, K., Dibb, L., Shenton, F., & Elson, N. (2001). No one's ever asked me: Young people with a prisoner in the family. Retrieved from http://www.prisonersfamilies.org.uk/uploadedFiles/2010_Publications_And_Resources/Noones_ever_asked_me.pdf

Children, Youth and Families Act. (2005). Retrieved from http://www.austlii.edu.au/

Chui, W. H. (2016). Voices of the incarcerated father: Struggling to live up to fatherhood. *Criminology and Criminal Justice*, 16(1), 60–79.

Crimes Act. (1958).

Dallaire, D., & Wilson, L. (2010). The relation of exposure to parental criminal activity, arrest, and sentencing to children's maladjustment. *Journal of Child and Family Studies*, 19, 404–418.

Dennison, S., & Smallbone, H. (2015). You can"t be much of anything from inside': The implications of imprisoned fathers' parental involvement and generative opportunities for children's wellbeing. In A. Eriksson, & C. Flynn (Eds.), *Special edition: Children of prisoners. Law in context* (pp. 61–85), 32. NSW: Federation Press.

Dennison, S., Smallbone, H., Stewart, A., Freiberg, K., & Teague, R. (2014). "My life is separated": An examination of the challenges and barriers to parenting for indigenous fathers in prison. *British Journal of Criminology*, 54(1), 1089–1108.

Dennison, S., Stewart, A., & Freiberg, K. (2013). A prevalence study of children with imprisoned fathers: Annual and lifetime estimates. *Australian Journal of Social Issues, 48*(3), 339–362.

Department of Health and Human Services, see DHHS

DHHS. (2012). *Protecting Children: Protocol between Department of Health and Human Services, Child Protection and Victoria Police.* http://www.dhs.vic.gov.au/__data/assets/pdf_file/0019/442603/Protecting-Children-CP-and-VicPol-protocol-2012.pdf

Flynn, C., Bartlett, T., Fernandez Arias, P., Evans, P., & Burgess, A. (2015). Responding to children when their parents are incarcerated: Exploring the responses in Victoria and New South Wales, Australia. In A. Eriksson, & C. Flynn (Eds.), *Special edition: Children of prisoners. Law in context)* (pp. 4–27), 32. NSW: Federation Press.

Flynn, C., Naylor, B., & Fernandez, P. (2015). Responding to the needs of children of parents arrested in Victoria, Australia: The role of the adult criminal justice system. *Australia and New Zealand Journal of Criminology, 0*(0). doi:10.1177/0004865815585390

Glaze, L. E., & Kaeble, D. (2014). *Correctional Populations in the United States*, 2013 (NCJ 248479). Retrieved from http://www.bjs.gov/index.cfm?ty=pbdetail&iid=5177

Glaze, L. E., & Maruschak, L. (2008). *Incarcerated parents and their minor children* (NCJ 222984). Retrieved from http://www.bjs.gov/content/pub/pdf/pptmc.pdf

Halsey, M., & Deegan, S. (2012). Father and son: Two generations through prison. *Punishment & Society, 14*(3), 338–367.

IACP. (2014). *Safeguarding children of arrested parents.* Retrieved from https://www.bja.gov/Publications/IACP-SafeguardingChildren.pdf

IACP. (2016). Safeguarding children of arrested parents. Retrieved from http://www.iacp.org/cap

International Association of Chiefs of Police, see IACP

Johnston, D., & Gabel, K. (1995). Incarcerated parents. In K. Gabel, & D. Johnston (Eds.), *Children of incarcerated parents* (pp. 3–20). New York, NY: Lexington Books.

Liamputtong, P. (2007). *Researching the vulnerable: A guide to sensitive research methods.* London: Sage Publications.

Lilburn, S. (2001). Arresting moments: Identifying risks for women and their children from the time of police arrest. *Alternative Law Journal, 26*(3), 115–118.

Meek, R. (2011). The possible selves of young fathers in prison. *Journal of Adolescence, 34*(5), 941–949.

Moran, D. (2017). "Daddy is a difficult word for me to hear": carceral geographies of parenting and the prison visiting room as a contested space of situated fathering. *Children's Geographies, 15*(1), 107–121.

Mulready-Jones, A. (2011). *Hidden children: A study into services for Children of Incarcerated Parents in Sweden and the United States.* Retrieved from http://www.wcmt.org.uk/sites/default/files/migrated-reports/814_1.pdf

Neville, K. (2010). Forgotten children: Law enforcement agencies, child protective services, and children of arrested parents in Michigan. *McNair Scholars Research Journal, 2*(1), 165–179.

Nieto, M. (2002). *In danger of falling through the cracks: Children of arrested parents.* California, CA: California Research Bureau.

Nurse, A. (2002). *Fatherhood arrested: Parenting from within the juvenile justice system.* Nashville, TN: Vanderbilt University Press.

Patton, M. Q. (2002). *Qualitative research and evaluation methods* (3rd ed.). Thousand Oaks, CA: Sage Publications.

Phillips, S. D., & Zhao, J. (2010). The relationship between witnessing arrests and elevated symptoms of posttraumatic stress: Findings from a national study of children involved in the child welfare system. *Children and Youth Services Review, 32*(1), 1246–1254.

Puddefoot, G., & Foster, L. K. (2007). *Keeping children safe when their parents are arrested: Local approaches that work.* Sacramento, CA: California Research Bureau.

Simmons, C. (2000). *Children of incarcerated parents.* Sacramento, CA: California Research Bureau.

The Pew Charitable Trusts. (2010). *Collateral costs: Incarceration's effects on economic mobility.* Retrieved from http://www.pewtrusts.org/~/media/legacy/uploadedfiles/pcs_assets/2010/collateralcosts1pdf.pdf

The Yale Child Study Center. (2011). Yale Child Study Center Trauma Section. Retrieved from http://medicine.yale.edu/childstudy/community/nccev.aspx

Trotter, C., Flynn, C., Naylor, B., Collier, P., Baker, D., McCauley, K., & Eriksson, A. (2015). *The impact of incarceration on children's care: A strategic framework for good care planning.* Melbourne: Monash University.

Victoria Police. (2013). *Victoria police annual report 2012–13.* Retrieved from http://www.police. vic.gov.au/content.asp?a=internetBridgingPage&Media_ID=97049

Victoria Police. (2014). *Crime Statistics 2013-14.* Retrieved from http://www.police.vic.gov.au/ crimestats/ebooks/1213/crimestats2012-13.pdf

Victoria Police. (2017). *Victoria Police Manual-Guidelines.* Victoria, AUS. Author Retrieved from file:///C:/Users/btess/Downloads/VPMG_SafeCustodyGuide_final.pdf.

Walmsley, R. (2016). *World prison population list, 11th edition.* Retrieved from: http://www. prisonstudies.org/sites/default/files/resources/downloads/world_prison_population_list_11th_ edition_0.pdf

Wright, L., & Seymour, B. (2000). *Working with children and families separated by incarceration: A handbook for child welfare agencies.* Washington, DC: CWLA Press.

The (Dis)continuity of Parenthood Among Incarcerated Fathers: An Analysis of Caregivers' Accounts

Melinda Tasca

ABSTRACT

The intersection of mass incarceration and fatherhood is of particular interest to a growing number of scholars, policymakers, and practitioners. In this study, the role of fathers in children's lives before and during imprisonment are investigated from the caregiver perspective. Reliance on caregivers' accounts offers valuable insight into the complexities of fathers' involvement with children prior to and during incarceration. Data come from the Arizona Children of Incarcerated Parents (COIP) project and rely on in-depth interviews with a diverse set of 53 caregivers of children, including mothers (current/former partners), grandparents, extended family, and non-relatives. Findings reveal that while slightly more than half of caregivers (58%, $n = 31$) reported involvement by fathers in the lives of children prior to prison, considerably more (81%, $n = 43$) reported contact between fathers and children during imprisonment. Thematic content analysis was conducted to explore key themes in caregivers' narratives to explain the continuity and disconnects in fatherhood. Overall, results highlight the need for intervention efforts that focus on incarcerated fathers and their children that are cognizant of variation in family life, as well as the central role of caregivers.

Introduction

Increasing scholarship highlights the broad-reaching effects of mass imprisonment on inmates, children, families, and communities (Arditti, 2012; National Research Council, 2014; Turanovic, Rodriguez, & Pratt, 2012). Despite evidence of declining prison populations in some jurisdictions, the incarceration rate in the United States remains significantly higher than the rest of the industrialized world (Carson & Anderson, 2016; Clear, 2007). This has resulted in incarceration becoming a normalized life event in the trajectories of predominately disadvantaged men in the U.S.—more than half of whom are fathers of minor children (Glaze & Maruschak, 2008; Turney, 2015a, 2015b). These fathers tend to suffer from an accumulation of stressors prior to incarceration including substance abuse, mental and physical health problems, low educational attainment, and underemployment (Arditti, Smock, & Parkman, 2005; Galardi, Settersten, Vuchinich, & Richards, 2017; Swisher & Waller, 2008). Material hardship and residential instability is also a common theme in their lives and in the lives of their families (Geller & Franklin, 2014; Tasca, Rodriguez, & Zatz, 2011; Wildeman, 2014). Incarcerated fathers are part of highly complicated family systems, in which relationships with their children's mothers and other caregivers are often fragile, as reflected by high rates of family conflict and relationship dissolution (Roy & Burton, 2007; Roy & Dyson, 2005; Tasca, Mulvey, & Rodriguez, 2016). Together, these dynamics and experiences pose significant challenges for fathering before and following incarceration.

Federal and state initiatives aimed at increasing responsible fatherhood have been in place in the U.S. for decades as a result of rising birth rates among poor, single parents (Lopoo & Raissian, 2014). Recent efforts have become increasingly visible to the general public through widespread campaigns that encourage fathers' engagement with their children, and even in political speeches, most notably by former President Obama, where he called upon young men to step up as fathers (Edin, Tach, & Mincy, 2009; see the National Responsible Fatherhood Clearinghouse, 2017). Entire bodies of literature have been devoted to fathering and its implications for children, family life, and society more broadly. Yet, much of this work and related interventions have not considered the intersection of imprisonment in the lives of these vulnerable families (Geller, 2013; Turney, 2015a; Wakefield & Wildeman, 2014). While this is beginning to change, critical gaps in knowledge remain in how fatherhood is shaped by incarceration (Rodriguez, 2016).

What is more, few studies have explored the nuances of incarcerated fathers' involvement through the lens of a wide range of caregivers who provide primary care for these children (i.e. mothers, grandparents, extended family members, non-relatives). These individuals play critical roles in the facilitation of contact between fathers and their children, especially during periods of confinement. Caregivers have been referred to as "gatekeepers" in that they are responsible for making decisions about children's best interests, including if, and how much contact, children have with incarcerated fathers (Roy & Dyson, 2005; Tasca, 2016). And for many families, these individuals have served in their current roles for most of the children's lives, making caregivers' perspectives central to understanding the impact of parental incarceration on family functioning and child well-being (Poehlmann, Dallaire, Loper, & Shear, 2010; Turanovic et al., 2012).

Accordingly, the purpose of this study is to explore the role of fathers in children's lives before and during imprisonment, using in-depth interviews with 53 caregivers in Arizona. Drawing on accounts of caregivers who represent diverse family systems can shed important light on the continuity and disconnects in father–child contact. In so doing, this study contributes to growing interdisciplinary work on incarcerated fatherhood and the consequences for children and family life, and also offers directions for policy and practice.

Background

The number of children born into poverty and to unmarried parents has led to an abundance of research on fathering and family functioning (Augustine, Nelson, & Edin, 2009; Edin et al., 2009; Lopoo & Raissian, 2014). Studies have documented how economic shifts from the 1950s through the most recent recession have affected patterns of relationship formation and family stability among disadvantaged populations (Edin & Nelson, 2013; Tach, Edin, Harvey, & Bryan, 2014). In recent decades, children have become more likely to be in the care of extended family as well—particularly grandparents—who serve as essential components of what Cherlin and Seltzer (2014) call the "family safety net."

In their influential work on fatherhood among low-income men, Edin and Nelson (2013) described a key shift in parenthood. For many vulnerable fathers interviewed in their study, infants were considered a "blessing" in the midst of constant struggle and fragile relationships. With parenthood, however, came expectations of responsibility and most of these men described difficulties in meeting the demands of conventional fatherhood. As such, they were left to "do the best they can" which entailed spending time with children when feasible and using their own lives as "cautionary tales." This study and others document increasing complexity in family life and the shifting roles of men as fathers and partners (Augustine et al., 2009; Edin et al., 2009; Roy & Burton, 2007).

Incarcerated fathers reflect an increasing segment of these men who are high in risk and need due to marginalization in family and economic spheres (Arditti et al., 2005; Turney, 2015b). These fathers are overwhelmingly poor, young, men of color, with low levels of education, and limited employment histories, which contribute to family and residential instability well before incarceration (National Research Council, 2014). U.S. national estimates indicate that the majority of incarcerated fathers lived apart from their children prior to involvement in the criminal justice system (Glaze & Maruschak, 2008). However, recent research shows that these men are often engaged in fathering in other ways, including visiting with their children, or providing material assistance (Dennison & Smallbone, 2015; Geller, 2013). Since incarceration has become an all too common experience in the lives of disadvantaged men, opportunities for father–child contact frequently exist from behind bars (Arditti, 2012; Swanson, Lee, Sansone, & Tatum, 2013). Indeed, Arditti and colleagues explain that, "one point at which fathers are increasingly located on the 'social radar screen' is behind the fence in correctional facilities" (Arditti et al., 2005, p. 269).

For many families, the confinement period represents a chance for a fresh slate with respect to fatherhood (Arditti et al., 2005; Tasca et al., 2016; Turney, 2015a). Fathers' beliefs that circumstances will improve—and by extension so will their relationships with their children—is widespread in the literature (Arditti et al., 2005; Day, Acock, Bahr, & Arditti, 2005). In fact, many fathers attempt to initiate or repair relationships with their children when they are behind bars (Roy & Dyson, 2005). This process is complicated, however, by the reality that fathers are dependent upon their children's caregivers to nurture that relationship. To be sure, these mothers, grandparents, extended family members, and friends are gatekeepers of fathers' relationships with children, especially during incarceration (Roy & Dyson, 2005; Tasca, 2016). Most decisions about contact with an incarcerated father are made by mothers or other caregivers rather than by a judge or social worker (Poehlmann et al., 2010). Thus, caregivers are in a pivotal position as they may enable communication, or prohibit contact altogether.

The literature on maternal gatekeeping in disrupted families suggests that while many factors are at play, relationship quality between parents is an important predictor of father–child contact (Edin et al., 2009; Fagan & Barnett, 2003). Evidence also indicates that mothers overwhelmingly promote and value father–child relationships (Roy & Dyson, 2005). When women restrict fathers' involvement, it is often due to questions surrounding paternal fitness (Fagan & Barnett, 2003; Swanson et al., 2013). It is important to note that histories of drug use, mental health problems, and longstanding involvement in crime characterize much of the inmate population (The National Research Council, 2014). These challenges can take a toll on relationships and stand in the way of parenting, especially if family members were victims of violence or abuse (Rodriguez, 2016). Approximately half of fathers in Roy and Dyson's (2005) study on maternal gatekeeping indicated that mothers restricted access to children during paternal incarceration. The extent to which limited access to fathers was beneficial for children, or simply due to barriers, is not clear, however (Arditti et al., 2005; Roy & Dyson, 2005). How gatekeeping behavior manifests among caregivers other than mothers is also poorly understood (Tasca, 2016).

There is some evidence to suggest that father–child contact increases and relationships are improved while a father is behind bars (Geller, 2013; Roy & Dyson, 2005; Turney, 2015a). During incarceration, many fathers may be finally sober, available, and attentive which leads to optimism among caregivers about their ability to contribute to children and family life (Tasca et al., 2016). Other research describes caregivers as empathetic to paternal incarceration, which opens the door to increased communication and contact with children (Roy & Dyson, 2005). In light of the desire for a father for children, some caregivers stand by these men despite their frustrations (Edin & Nelson, 2013; Roy & Burton, 2007; Tasca, 2016). To be certain, stories of men earning "second chances" flow through much of this work (Roy & Burton, 2007; Turney, 2015b). For others, prolonged unemployment, abuse, and addiction led to the severing of ties well before any period of confinement (Geller, 2013; Turanovic et al., 2012). While scholarship has started to tap into the variability in family life among those experiencing incarceration (Rodriguez, 2016; Scharff Smith, 2014), much remains to be learned about paternal involvement patterns and the role of caregivers in the process.

Current study

In an effort to contribute to scholarship on the collateral consequences of imprisonment and the policy dialog surrounding the state of fatherhood, this study investigates the role of fathers in the lives of children before and during imprisonment from the caregiver perspective. Data come from the Arizona Children of Incarcerated Parents Project (COIP) and rely on in-depth interviews with 53 caregivers of children including mothers, grandparents, extended family, and non-relatives. Exploring the (dis)continuity of fathering through this lens offers important insights for research, policy, and practice.

Data and method

These data come from the COIP, which was a two-phase project carried out between 2010 and 2011. The first phase of data collection involved the completion of structured interviews with 300 men incarcerated in the Arizona Department of Corrections (ADC) who self-identified as being the parent of at least one minor child.[1] As part of the protocol, incarcerated fathers were asked if they were willing to provide contact information for their children's caregivers so that researchers could interview these individuals about their experiences as well. Interviews with caregivers comprised the second phase of the project, which generated the data analyzed in this paper.

In-depth interviews were conducted with 53 caregivers of children of incarcerated fathers. Researchers recruited caregivers through phone calls and letters using contact information provided from incarcerated fathers interviewed during the first phase of the project.[2] Participation was voluntary and caregivers received $50 for their participation in a 60 to 90-minute interview. Nearly all interviews were conducted in private, university offices. For some participants, however, commuting to campus was not feasible due to lack of transportation or physical ailments. In an effort to accommodate these caregivers, a researcher conducted phone interviews in lieu of face-to-face meetings. All interviews were recorded and later transcribed by a professional transcriptionist.

Caregiver interviews provided rich descriptions about various aspects of families' lives before and during a father's incarceration. Researchers relied on an interview protocol comprised of open-ended questions which allowed probing of participants' responses. Interviews focused on multiple domains, including caregiver perceptions of parent–child contact, relationship dynamics, living situations, as well as social support, child well-being, and family service needs. As demonstrated by prior work, incarcerated fathers' involvement with children is often nuanced and intertwined with complicated relationships with children's mothers and other caregivers (Arditti et al., 2005; Roy & Burton, 2007; Roy & Dyson, 2005). Thus, reliance on detailed caregiver accounts offers valuable insight into the complexities of fathers' involvement with children before and during paternal incarceration.

With respect to sample characteristics, the majority of caregivers were mothers of children. Approximately 28% of the 53 caregivers were mothers/current partners, 41% were mothers/former partners, 23% were grandparents, and 8% were other relatives or friends. Caregivers were racially and ethnically diverse (i.e. White = 21%, Black = 36%, Latino/a = 26%, Native American = 17%). Only 6% of caregivers were male. The average age was 36, although caregivers spanned from 18 to 74 years old. The number of children ranged from one to six, with a mean of two children in care. Finally, 70% of caregivers reported receiving public assistance during interviews.

Interview transcripts were reviewed and first coded according to fathers' involvement before incarceration (i.e. involved or uninvolved/limited involvement). "Prior parental involvement" reflected fathers who were reported by caregivers as having either (a) lived with, (b) had visits or substantive interactions with, and/or (c) provided tangible support for their children before imprisonment (e.g. material items, informal or formal financial support). "No involvement" consisted of fathers who were reported by caregivers to have been completely absent in all respects, while "limited involvement" reflected fathers who had at least met their children, but had minimal presence in their lives, and did not provide tangible support for them prior to confinement. Cases where caregivers indicated no or limited involvement were collapsed into a single category in analysis.

The author then coded transcripts for fathers' involvement during incarceration. This was captured by whether there was prison contact between children and fathers since confinement (i.e. visits, phone calls, letters). These coding procedures resulted in the following typologies: (1) Previously involved fathers who: (a) had contact with their children during incarceration; and (b) those who no longer had any contact with children since incarceration. And, (2) previously uninvolved fathers who: (a) did have contact with their children while in prison; and (b) those who continued to have no contact at all. Thematic content analysis was conducted to explore key themes in caregivers' narratives to explain the (dis)-continuity in fatherhood before and during imprisonment across these typologies (Lofland & Lofland, 1995). Descriptive background characteristics were also compiled to provide further information on these groups.

Findings

Roughly 58% ($n = 31$) of caregivers reported involvement by fathers in the lives of children prior to imprisonment, while 42% ($n = 22$) of caregivers indicated there was no (or very limited) prior paternal involvement. Yet, 81% ($n = 43$) of caregivers reported prison contact between fathers and children (visits only = 16%; phone calls only = 9%; letters only = 16%; and multiple forms of contact = 59%). Only 19% ($n = 10$) of caregivers reported no father–child contact during incarceration (Table 1).

Interesting patterns emerged regarding the (dis)continuity of involvement before and during paternal incarceration. Among the 31 caregivers who reported prior father involvement, 90% ($n = 28$) described contact between fathers and children during imprisonment. That is, only 10% ($n = 3$) of fathers who were previously involved with their children had no prison contact, according to caregivers. Among the 22 caregivers who reported no/very limited prior paternal involvement, 68% ($n = 15$) described prison contact between fathers and children, while 32% ($n = 7$) of caregivers reported no prison contact. To explain these disconnects in father–child contact before and during imprisonment, key themes uncovered through thematic content analysis are discussed below.

Table 1. Summary of Father Involvement Patterns before and during Incarceration.

	Prior Involvement	Prior Non-Involvement
Prison Contact	28	15
No Prison Contact	3	7

Note. $N = 53$ caregivers.

Prior father involvement: ongoing contact

As previously mentioned, 90% ($n = 28$) of the 31 caregivers who reported prior involvement by fathers indicated there was contact between fathers and children during imprisonment. Most of these caregivers were children's mothers and current partners of the incarcerated fathers (39%). A sizeable portion, however, were also former partners (21%). More than one-quarter of these caregivers were children's grandparents and 11% were other family members or friends. This set of caregivers and incarcerated fathers were disproportionately African American (46% and 54% respectively). One-third of incarcerated fathers in this group were convicted of violent offenses, and the same proportion were convicted of drug and property crimes. The average prison term was 57 months. Despite these fathers' prior involvement in their children's lives, roughly half had served time in prison previously.

Father–child contact supports child well-being

Two major themes emerged from the narratives of this group of caregivers. The first centered on the importance of maintaining a father–child relationship for child well-being. Importantly, this set of families was characterized as having the closest relationships with fathers. While caregivers certainly described "ups and downs" in their family relationships and circumstances—and some were uncomfortable with what prison contact entailed—caregivers expressed that disruption in paternal involvement could lead to adverse outcomes for children. One caregiver, a Latina grandmother, explained how paternal imprisonment and the process of maintaining contact was challenging for her grandchild. That said, she found through continued contact, not only is the relationship between her son and grandson strengthened, her grandson benefitted emotionally and behaviorally from the guidance his father provided. She also found the father's enforcement of rules and boundaries helpful, even during incarceration:

> It was irritating at first because the kids shouldn't have to deal with this. But the positive side is that he gets to still bond with his father. If he didn't, [my grandson] would have more issues. It also helps me because [the father] gives [his son] advice and backs me on things I'm trying to follow through with him on.

Another caregiver, a Black mother and current partner of the incarcerated father, discussed her views of traditional gender roles in parenting. From her standpoint, the continuation of their co-parenting strategy during the father's imprisonment helped their adolescent son avoid problem behaviors:

> A mom is like really passive when you grow up, but a Dad is like "get over there, and do what you're supposed to do, do what your Mom said … " I don't know it all. I can't teach him to be a man. Without that contact, I would probably have a problem.

For many, family life before the father's incarceration was far from smooth. Caregivers described dealing with paternal drug use, involvement in child welfare, and intimate partner violence at the hands of some of these men. To be sure, this group had the highest proportion of involvement with child protective services, with one in five caregivers reporting that these children were involved with CPS at some point in their lives. This group also had the highest rates of paternal substance abuse, in which 79% of fathers were described as having problems with drugs and/or alcohol. In addition, 11% of caregivers indicated that they had been the victim of abuse and/or violence by the incarcerated father. Nonetheless, for this group, having a relationship with one's father was seen by caregivers as invaluable and considered independent of any past wrongdoings. Based on caregivers' own personal experiences, they believed these children would suffer in the short- and long-term without their fathers in their lives. This perspective is reflected in the following narrative of one mother, who separated the tumultuous history and intimate partner violence she experienced at the hands of her former boyfriend and children's father from his role as "dad":

> I read that girls who grow up without dads end up in bad relationships. I think that's why I ended up in the relationship I did, and of course, withstood it for so long because I didn't have my dad to raise me and to tell me "okay, this is not right" and stuff like that. I think that it did affect me a lot so that's my concern with my daughters is that they're gonna be in the same position. That's why I push for him to be in their lives so much so they're not out looking for love or something, you know what I mean? (Mother, Former Partner, Latina).

In a separate account, a grandmother—whose grandchildren were placed with her by the state prior to the father's incarceration as a result of parental neglect and drug abuse—explained that maintaining a connection to their incarcerated father was in the children's best interests:

> Right before their father was incarcerated, both of the parents were on drugs. Their mother more so than their father, and they just lived in unhealthy conditions. Child Protective Services took [the kids] away and I asked if I could have them. Even with all that, [the kids] still need to have a relationship with their father (Grandmother, White).

Families need to "stick together"

The second theme emphasizes the need for families to "stick together." Since fathers were consistently involved in these children's day-to-day lives before imprisonment, forgiveness and moving forward together was central for these families. Caregivers described how it was critical to continue to support one another, even though "mistakes" were made:

> I don't want [my son] to think that his father loves him any less because he made a mistake. I want him to always know his father. His father's not a bad person (Mother, Current Partner, White).

> I view [contact] as a positive thing. I was happy he got to see his babies. Nothing negative about that. Just because a father goes to jail that doesn't mean you gotta give up. Basically, just don't give up (Mother, Former Partner, Black).

> I wouldn't abandon him. That's not the type of person I am. Like, whatever we go through, the kids are always his … I would rather them have a dad (Mother, Current Partner, Black).

One caregiver described an exchange he had with his niece and nephew who he had been caring for since their father's incarceration. For him, and others in this group, showing support to fathers during incarceration was an attempt at both securing success in re-entry and family reunification:

> I explained to them, "Okay, by you guys going to see him, it's out of support. That gives him strength to survive through that so that he can make it back to you. By me taking you guys up there, that lets him know that I'm gonna be loyal, and make sure that when he does get out, I can get him on the right track so he doesn't go back" (Uncle, Black).

Taken together, despite past adversities, continuity in father involvement (and family life more broadly) was the top priority for this set of families.

Prior father involvement: no prison contact

A small number of fathers were also involved in children's lives before incarceration, but had not had any contact since imprisonment. This subset of families comprised just three cases, of the 31 with prior paternal contact. These caregivers were mothers of the children—two mothers were current partners and one was a former partner of the fathers. They had a higher number of children relative to other groups (i.e. three children, on average) and their children were also younger (i.e. average age of the youngest child in care was 18 months). Two of these caregivers and incarcerated fathers were Latino/a and one caregiver and incarcerated father was African American. Two men were incarcerated for drug offenses, while one was in prison for violent crime. Only one of the three men had been in prison before. Yet, they were serving substantially longer sentences than other incarcerated fathers, with an average prison term of 144 months. These familial relationships were characterized as more strained than close which was mostly attributed to the fathers' imprisonment, according to caregivers. No child protective service involvement or victimization by these fathers was reported; although two of these fathers were characterized by caregivers as having a history of mental illness.

Institutional and personal barriers to contact

The narratives of these women revealed a desire for their children to have contact with their previously involved fathers but life circumstances and institutional barriers prevented it. Following the father's incarceration, all of the women experienced increased hardship and residential instability. Two of the women reported receiving multiple forms of public assistance. This accumulation of challenges made having any contact—visits, phone calls, or letters—difficult. One of the mothers described how navigating the challenges of daily life was her sole priority:

> I was almost homeless. Then my one-year-old was hospitalized for months. He was really, really sick. I went into a big depression cause he was on life support and I didn't know what to do. No transportation. That was hard. My attention was just on my son and kids (Mother, Current Partner, Latina).

Another mother explained how her financial struggles prevented contact at first, but then, she decided that she and her children should simply move on in light of the father's lengthy prison sentence:

> I didn't have the money for calls, or to get out there and visit, or have transportation. As time went by, I kind of just let it go. Try to move on with my life, be strong for my kids. Can't hold on to something that's not there (Mother, Former Partner, Black).

Each of these women discussed barriers to contact including needing proper identification, the application process for calls and visits, and the expenses involved. Given how young their children were, and how frequently they were moving, there were barriers to written contact too. While all caregivers discussed barriers to contact to some extent, these women were either unable to overcome them, focused on other demands, and/or simply decided it was best that the family discontinue a relationship with the incarcerated father altogether.

Prior non-involvement by fathers: prison contact

The next set of findings focuses on families with previously uninvolved fathers. To reiterate, 42% ($n = 22$) of the 53 caregivers in the full sample reported no (or very limited) prior father involvement. Yet, 68% ($n = 15$) of these caregivers reported that there was father–child contact during incarceration. Among this group, 60% of caregivers were former partners and also children's mothers. Thirteen percent were mothers and current partners, 20% were grandparents, and 7% were other family or friends. These caregivers had the oldest children in their care (i.e. 10 years was the average age of the oldest child in care). With respect to the racial/ethnic composition of this group, Native Americans were overrepresented (i.e. 33% of caregivers and 13% of incarcerated fathers were Native American) and nearly three-fourths of these caregivers received public assistance.

Fathers were equally incarcerated for violent (40%) and drug offenses (40%) and were serving average prison terms of 56 months.

Second chance fathering

Not surprisingly, these familial relationships were quite strained. At the same time, narratives revealed the value placed on second chance fathering. That is, a father's imprisonment opened the door for *initiating* a relationship between children and their previously uninvolved fathers. As one mother and former partner (White) described, "Being in prison made [his father] consistently involved; with visits, obviously he was there. That was the only good thing that came from his incarceration." Another caregiver—a Native American grandfather—explained that since his son was incarcerated, "He calls his daughters three times a week. It's like he is right there. It is very important that they get to know their dad." Most caregivers were skeptical about whether fathers' engagement with their children would last given prior histories, however. Sixty percent of these previously uninvolved fathers were described by caregivers as having a history of substance abuse and 40% had been in prison before. The following narrative showcases a common sentiment expressed by caregivers:

> He sends them letters and he tries to be a positive role model *now* but they're gonna have their own opinion when he gets out. I don't want to put things in their head so I don't say anything, but I don't think he's gonna change. He will be the same person he was and they're gonna want their dad regardless. But they will see that he's still stuck in his ways (Mother, Former Partner, White).

Another mother explained that despite her own tumultuous history with her children's father, his lack of involvement, and extensive incarceration record, she was hopeful that it wasn't too late for him to begin a relationship with their adolescent children while in prison:

> He was abusive. I was abused by him the whole time I was with him and he wasn't helping me. It has been really, really rough. This last incarceration, he called me up and says, "well, I gotta go do three years," and I was like, "are you kidding me?" But I'm giving him a chance to be a father to his kids. It's just about being there for the kids (Mother, Former Partner, Black).

Seven percent of this set of caregivers reported a history of violence or abuse by the incarcerated father and 13% indicated that the children had been involved with child protective services. One grandmother shared how her grandson was a newborn when his father was most recently incarcerated. She was the primary guardian, but her daughter (the child's mother) takes the young boy to visit his father in prison in an effort to grow a father–child bond:

> [My grandson] knows who his dad is. He calls him dad and stuff. I think every child should know their parents, period. I mean, if it's in prison, if it's wherever. [His father] will be thirty-some years old [when he gets out] and I hope he gets it through his head, you know. Hopefully he gets on the right foot (Grandmother, Latina).

While remaining cautiously optimistic, this family—like many others—was committed to using the incarceration period to establish a father–child relationship that was missing before.

Prior non-involvement by fathers: no prison contact

Among the 22 caregivers in the full sample who reported no (or very limited) prior paternal involvement, 32% ($n = 7$) indicated that no father–child contact continued during imprisonment. This set of caregivers was comprised of the largest portion of former partners/children's mothers (86%) and the remaining caregivers were grandparents (14%). Caregivers and incarcerated fathers in this group were disproportionately White (57% and 43% respectively). This group also had the highest rate of public assistance, with 86% of caregivers reporting receipt of government aid. These families had highly strained relationships with incarcerated fathers and nearly one-third of caregivers described these relationships as "non-existent." These caregivers also reported the highest rate of prior victimization by incarcerated fathers (14%) and a similar portion reported that children had a history of child protective service involvement. While 70% of fathers were reported by caregivers to suffer from substance abuse problems, none of these caregivers reported mental health problems among fathers. Violent offenders were also overrepresented, with 58% of fathers incarcerated for violent crime. These men were serving average prison terms of 65 months; nearly three-quarters had been imprisoned previously, the highest proportion of all groups.

No contact is in the children's best interests

According to these caregivers, no contact with fathers was in the best interests of their children. While all families experienced stressors, this group was unique in some of the adversities they faced. As previously mentioned, this set of incarcerated fathers had particularly lengthy histories of incarceration and violence. These caregivers were entrenched in various public systems; and they, along with their children, experienced longstanding strained and non-existent relationships with incarcerated fathers. Put simply, these families had "had enough." The narrative below illustrates this view, while also recognizing the complex emotions surrounding no father–child contact:

> Well, he started using drugs, and became incarcerated again soon after [my daughter's] birth. I wondered, would it be the best thing just to completely cut him off? I hated to do that, but as a mom, you know, it's my duty, it's my job to do what's best for my daughter and there were always so many let downs (Mother, Former Partner, White).

The following caregiver described how she and her children had become fed up with the father's empty promises of being "a dad" while continuing to cycle in and out of correctional facilities:

> He was always going in and out of jail and out of their lives. Just not being there as a dad. My kids don't want to see him. He gotta come out and prove that he wants to see his kids and in the right way. Cause when you're in jail you make a lot of promises: "I'm gonna change" and when they get out it's the same old … I want better for my kids. I don't want negative people around them because they are already going through so much (Mother, Former Partner, Black).

She further expressed how her focus was not on the absence of her children's father, but rather on the maintenance of close relationships with extended family upon whom they rely for instrumental and emotional support. Another caregiver shared how her former partner's abusive history led to no contact with his children:

> I always wanted that house wife thing. With the kids' dad, together like a family, and have a white picket fence. No. It couldn't happen. I ended up pregnant again and living at his house at the time, and he was very abusive to me. I drew ourselves away and then later he went to prison. We didn't do wrong. He did. I don't think my kids should have to suffer and go sit there and visit him. We send no pictures. No contact has been going on for six and a half years (Mother, Former Partner, Latina).

This caregiver maintained that contact would be harmful to her children's well-being. While this group of caregivers discussed the importance of a father for their children, they did not foresee these particular men as able or willing to fulfill that role.

Discussion

This study explored the (dis)continuity in father involvement before and during incarceration, drawing upon the perspective of a diverse set of caregivers. Similar to other estimates of disadvantaged father engagement, 58% ($n = 31$) of caregivers reported prior father involvement (Dennison & Smallbone, 2015; Geller, 2013). Among this subset of families, nearly all (90%; $n = 28$) maintained father–child contact during paternal imprisonment. Among families with previously uninvolved fathers (42%; $n = 22$), more than two-thirds of caregivers reported that there was contact between fathers and children while in prison ($n = 15$). On balance, these patterns are consistent with other work that suggests children's accessibility to fathers can actually increase during paternal incarceration (Geller, 2013; Roy & Dyson, 2005; Turney, 2015a). These findings also speak more broadly to intergenerational trends of marginality among disadvantaged fathers, in which these men are largely sequestered from mainstream social, domestic, and economic life (Turney, 2015b). Incarceration, a normalized experience for many vulnerable families, represents a rare opportunity to build, maintain, or repair often fragile father–child relationships. As one caregiver explained, "Being in prison made [him] consistently involved; with visits, obviously he was there."

Thematic content analysis was also conducted to better understand reasons for these patterns. The first group included families with previously involved fathers who were also in contact with children during incarceration. In line with prior work, caregivers expressed that continued contact was necessary for child well-being and also noted the importance of "sticking together" as a family (Arditti et al., 2005; Roy & Burton, 2007). While familial relationships were characterized as close, these fathers, caregivers, and children experienced many stressors. To be sure, these families had the highest rates of caregiver-reported paternal substance abuse and involvement in child protective services. Black caregivers and fathers were also overrepresented. Research suggests that high rates of criminal justice system involvement among Black males has lessened the stigma of their incarceration and has also altered the ways in which parenting roles are enacted and accepted (Swisher & Waller, 2008; Tach et al., 2014). Overall, these patterns are reflective of other studies that describe caregivers' desires to achieve the "gold standard" of family life—one that they themselves yearned to have growing up (Edin & Nelson, 2013; Roy & Burton, 2007). While family members described having been let down along the way, many articulated that some paternal involvement is better than none at all.

The second group, comprised of families with fathers who were previously involved but had no contact with children since imprisonment, was small. This points to the continuity of contact for most men who were engaged with their children before confinement. Institutional barriers and material hardship were cited by these mothers as reasons for lack of contact (Swanson et al., 2013; Tasca, 2016). At the same time, as with Turney's work on romantic relationships of incarcerated men (2015a, 2015b), the confinement period provided some women and their young children freedom and opportunity to move forward with their lives.

The third group focused on fathers who were uninvolved with their children before incarceration, yet had contact during confinement. Key themes underlying this disconnect in father–child contact included caregivers' beliefs in second chances and the viewing of incarceration as an opportunity to initiate parental relationships. Consistent with prior research, caregivers were cautiously optimistic about future paternal involvement given difficult histories (Roy & Burton, 2007). This pattern of discontinuity in contact further points to critical gaps in social support and the normalization of the carceral experience itself among some families affected by imprisonment (Geller & Franklin, 2014; Turney, 2015b). Interestingly, caregivers actively separated their experiences and perceptions of these men as partners, sons, and relatives from how they viewed their role as fathers. This dissonance might open the door to "idealized expectations" that have been documented in other studies on incarcerated parenthood (Day et al., 2005; Tasca et al., 2016). The extent to which fathering will continue outside the confines of the prison setting remains an open question for this group. The overrepresentation of Native Americans is also noteworthy and should be probed in future research.

There was continuity in the lack of contact among the fourth and final group. These fathers were described as uninvolved prior to prison, with no father–child contact since imprisonment. This set of families was unique in the accumulation of stressors they experienced. These caregivers reported the highest rate of victimization by fathers and the vast majority of these men were in prison for violent crime. Family relationships were highly strained given entrenchment in poverty, various public systems, and fathers cycling in and out of incarceration. Former partners and Whites were overrepresented. Patterns here are consistent with some work on maternal gatekeeping which suggests that father–child contact is highly dependent upon the quality of the relationship between parents (Fagan & Barnett, 2003; Roy & Dyson, 2005). Other research shows that White caregivers are the least likely to trust an incarcerated individual as a parent (Swisher & Waller, 2008; Woldoff & Washington, 2008). An accumulation of stressors, coupled with the long-term absence of these men as fathers, led many caregivers in this group to believe that children were better off without them. Emergent themes emulate growing scholarship on the variability in family outcomes resulting from parental absence (Turanovic et al., 2012; Turney, 2015b). That is, father non-involvement and incarceration may actually benefit some children and families (e.g. those who experience violence or abuse).

An overarching takeaway from this study is that most caregivers desired father involvement, with the majority reporting contact between incarcerated fathers and children. Although many fathers lived apart from their children before incarceration, they were often involved in other ways including providing care and material support (Dennison & Smallbone, 2015; Woldoff & Washington, 2008). Research on the collateral consequences of imprisonment has documented how children of incarcerated parents tend to experience a host of emotional, behavioral, structural, and economic challenges in their lives (Geller & Franklin, 2014; Scharff Smith, 2014; Tasca et al., 2011; Wakefield & Wildeman, 2014; Wildeman, 2014). Prison contact has been shown to minimize some of the harms associated with parental absence due to incarceration (Galardi et al., 2017; Poehlmann et al., 2010). Even children whose fathers were previously absent can benefit from the establishment or repair of paternal relationships through the receipt of guidance, support, and resources (Geller, 2013). In other cases, particularly those in which fathers were violent or otherwise harmful, no contact may be in children's best interests, however (Rodriguez, 2016; Turanovic et al., 2012).

Despite valuable insights gleaned from this work, there are limitations that should be acknowledged. In particular, this research relied on the accounts of 53 caregivers in one jurisdiction, and did not include perspectives of fathers or their children. This study also did not evaluate the quality or frequency of father–child contact. Additional research is needed that expands upon measures of parental involvement, drawing from multiple viewpoints and methodologies. Future work should also explore how children fare in response to varied patterns of father involvement before, during, and after incarceration.

Conclusion

As large numbers of disadvantaged men experience incarceration and fatherhood, policy-makers and practitioners confront complex challenges in promoting paternal involvement and child and family well-being. It is essential that policies focused on increasing incarcerated father engagement take into account the complexity of the family systems in which these men are embedded (Rodriguez, 2016). Intervention efforts must include caregivers beyond custodial mothers and recognize caregivers' role as decision-makers in the family (Tasca et al., 2016; Turanovic et al., 2012). While some families remain intact through imprisonment, other fathers meet their children in prison for the first time. Some families lose contact during incarceration due in part to institutional and financial barriers, whereas others simply want to move on with their lives. For some caregivers, a father's absence before and during incarceration was considered a good thing. Policies that push for increased father–child contact, without attention to varying needs and desires of family members, are unlikely to be effective (Rodriguez, 2016). As articulated by Arditti et al. (2005), at the very minimum, these policies should "do no harm."

The facilitation of father involvement in ways that benefit the family are critical. One promising avenue is through prison visitation as the incarceration period provides an opportunity for a fresh slate for many families. Structuring visitation to include child-friendly spaces and easing barriers to contact can increase visiting opportunities as well as improve the quality of interactions for families who desire relationships with incarcerated fathers (Arditti, 2012; Poehlmann et al., 2010). In addition, intervention efforts targeting incarcerated fathers and their families should focus on improving parenting skills, strengthening relationships, and managing expectations, as well as teaching healthy coping and communication strategies (Tasca, 2016). Co-parenting resources extended to a diverse range of caregivers during and following incarceration could also prove fruitful

(Rodriguez, 2016). More broadly, investments that create economic opportunities for the incarcerated and their families and also address needs related to substance abuse and mental health are vital for increasing responsible fathering, family stability, and disengagement from crime (Edin & Nelson, 2013; Roy & Burton, 2007; Tach et al., 2014). These recommendations, while ambitious, are important steps toward improving paternal engagement and the overall functioning of families affected by mass imprisonment.

Notes

1. Incarcerated fathers were interviewed at the state's central intake facility which allowed for the sampling of inmates across all security levels (i.e. minimum, medium, close, and maximum custody) and offense types. All male inmates are initially housed in ASPC Alhambra Reception pending security classification (which spans days/weeks). The only exclusion of inmates in this study were maximum security sex offenders as correctional staff did not permit interviewing of these offenders for safety reasons. Maximum security sex offenders, however, are a small portion of the male inmate population in ADC (less than 5%). Researchers were provided with a current count sheet of all inmates in the facility on a daily basis. From that list, every ninth prisoner was identified and subsequently approached by a member of the research team. Correctional staff did not screen or recruit inmates for participation in the study. Researchers would determine eligibility (i.e. whether the inmate reported being a parent of a child under the age of 18) and obtain consent. Interviews took place at tables in a designated area of the unit which ensured confidentiality. Per ADC policy, inmates were not permitted to receive incentives for taking part in interviews. The participation rate of approached and eligible inmates was 96%. This research was approved by the Institutional Review Board (IRB) at Arizona State University.
2. Given resource limitations, the sample included only caregivers with children residing in one large Arizona county. A random sample of 75 incarcerated fathers, with home addresses in this County, was compiled from the full sample of 300 fathers. Among those 75 paternal incarceration cases, 16 had a disconnected phone number or an invalid/incorrect number. Two caregivers did not respond to contact attempts, and two other caregivers declined participation in the study. Two interviews were conducted in Spanish but were excluded from the present study as they were not professionally transcribed.

Disclosure statement

No potential conflict of interest was reported by the author.

References

Arditti, J. A. (2012). *Parental incarceration and the family: Psychological and social effects of imprisonment on children, parents, and caregivers*. New York, NY: New York University Press.

Arditti, J. A., Smock, S. A., & Parkman, T. S. (2005). "It's been hard to be a father": A qualitative exploration of incarcerated fatherhood. *Fathering: A Journal of Theory, Research, and Practice About Men as Fathers, 3*(3), 267–288.

Augustine, J. M., Nelson, T., & Edin, K. (2009). Why do poor men have children? Fertility intentions among low-income unmarried U.S. fathers. *The ANNALS of the American Academy of Political and Social Science, 624*(1), 99–117.

Carson, A. E., & Anderson, E. (2016). *Prisoners in 2015.* (Report No. NCJ 250229). Washington, DC: U.S. Department of Justice, Bureau of Justice Statistics.

Cherlin, A. J., & Seltzer, J. A. (2014). Family complexity, the family safety net, and public policy. *The ANNALS of the American Academy of Political and Social Science, 654*(1), 231–239.

Clear, T. R. (2007). *Imprisoning communities: How mass incarceration makes disadvantaged neighborhoods worse.* New York: Oxford University Press.

Day, R. D., Acock, A. C., Bahr, S. J., & Arditti, J. A. (2005). Incarcerated fathers returning home to children and families: Introduction to the special issue and a primer on doing research with Men in prison. *Fathering: A Journal of Theory, Research, and Practice About Men as Fathers, 3*(3), 183–200.

Dennison, S., & Smallbone, H. (2015). "You can't be much of anything from inside": The implications of imprisoned fathers' parental involvement and generative opportunities for children's wellbeing. *Law in Context, 32*(1), 61–86.

Edin, K., & Nelson, T. J. (2013). *Doing the best I can: Fatherhood in the inner city.* Berkeley, CA: University of California Press.

Edin, K., Tach, L., & Mincy, R. (2009). Claiming fatherhood: Race and the dynamics of paternal involvement among unmarried men. *The Annals of the American Academy of Political and Social Science, 621*(1), 149–177.

Fagan, J., & Barnett, M. (2003). The relationship between maternal gatekeeping, paternal competence, mothers' attitudes about the father role, and father involvement. *Journal of Family Issues, 24*(8), 1020–1043.

Galardi, T. R., Settersten, R. A., Vuchinich, S., & Richards, L. (2017). Associations between incarcerated fathers' cumulative childhood risk and contact with their children. *Journal of Family Issues, 38*(5), 654–676.

Geller, A. (2013). Paternal incarceration and father-child contact in fragile families. *Journal of Marriage and Family, 75*(5), 1288–1303.

Geller, A., & Franklin, A. W. (2014). Paternal incarceration and the housing security of urban mothers. *Journal of Marriage and Family, 76*(2), 411–427.

Glaze, L. E., & Maruschak, L. M. (2008). *Parents in prison and their minor children.* (Report No. NCJ 222984). Washington, DC: U.S. Department of Justice, Bureau of Justice Statistics.

Lofland, J., & Lofland, L. H. (1995). *Analyzing social settings: A guide to qualitative observations and analysis.* Belmont, CA: Wadsworth.

Lopoo, L. M., & Raissian, K. M. (2014). U.S. social policy and family complexity. *The ANNALS of the American Academy of Political and Social Science, 654*(1), 213–230.

National Research Council. (2014). *The growth of incarceration in the United States: Exploring causes and consequences.* Committee on Causes and Consequences of High Rates of Incarceration. Washington, DC: The National Academies Press.

National Responsible Fatherhood Clearinghouse. (2017). Retrieved from https://www.fatherhood.gov/

Poehlmann, J., Dallaire, D., Loper, A. B., & Shear, L. D. (2010). Children's contact with their incarcerated parents: Research findings and recommendations. *American Psychologist, 65*(6), 575–598.

Rodriguez, N. (2016). Bridging the gap between research and practice. *The ANNALS of the American Academy of Political and Social Science, 665*(1), 231–240.

Roy, K., & Burton, L. (2007). Mothering through recruitment: Kinscription of nonresidential fathers and father figures in low-income families. *Family Relations, 56*(1), 24–39.

Roy, K., & Dyson, O. (2005). Gatekeeping in context: Babymama drama and the involvement of incarcerated fathers. *Fathering: A Journal of Theory, Research, and Practice About Men as Fathers, 3*(3), 289–310.

Scharff Smith, P. (2014). *When the innocent are punished: The children of incarcerated parents.* London: Palgrave Macmillan.

Swanson, C., Lee, C.-B., Sansone, F. A., & Tatum, K. M. (2013). Incarcerated fathers and their children: Perceptions of barriers to their relationships. *The Prison Journal, 93*(4), 453–474.

Swisher, R. R., & Waller, M. R. (2008). Confining fatherhood: Incarceration and paternal involvement among nonresident white, African American and Latino fathers. *Journal of Family Issues, 29*, 1067–1088.

Tach, L., Edin, K., Harvey, H., & Bryan, B. (2014). The family-go-round: Family complexity and father involvement from a father's perspective. *The ANNALS of the American Academy of Political and Social Science, 654*(1), 169–184.

Tasca, M. (2016). The gatekeepers of contact: Child-caregiver dyads and parental prison visitation. *Criminal Justice and Behavior, 43*(6), 739–758.

Tasca, M., Mulvey, P., & Rodriguez, N. (2016). Families coming together in prison: An examination of visitation encounters. *Punishment & Society, 18*(4), 459–478.

Tasca, M., Rodriguez, N., & Zatz, M. S. (2011). Family and residential instability in the context of paternal and maternal incarceration. *Criminal Justice and Behavior, 38*, 231–247.

Turanovic, J. J., Rodriguez, N., & Pratt, T. C. (2012). The collateral consequences of incarceration revisited: A qualitative analysis of the effects on caregivers of children of incarcerated parents. *Criminology, 50*(4), 913–959.

Turney, K. (2015a). Hopelessly devoted? Relationship quality during and after incarceration. *Journal of Marriage and Family, 77*(2), 480–495.

Turney, K. (2015b). Liminal Men: Incarceration and relationship dissolution. *Social Problems, 62* (4), 499–528.

Wakefield, S., & Wildeman, C. (2014). *Children of the prison boom: Mass incarceration and the future of American inequality.* New York: Oxford University Press.

Wildeman, C. (2014). Parental incarceration, child homelessness, and the invisible consequences of mass imprisonment. *The ANNALS of the American Academy of Political and Social Science, 651* (1), 74–96.

Woldoff, R. A., & Washington, H. M. (2008). Arrested contact: The criminal justice system, race, and father engagement. *The Prison Journal, 88*(2), 179–206.

Developing a Child's Right to Effective Contact with a Father in Prison—An Irish Perspective

Aisling Parkes and Fiona Donson

ABSTRACT

Recent years have witnessed a gradual increase in international research on the effects of parental incarceration on families and prisoners both in the short, medium and long term. However, the rights of children with a parent in prison is a subject which, in the Irish context at least, has been ill considered to date by policy and law makers. Research has shown that the consequences of failing to support this group of children can be adverse, not only for children concerned, but also for families and society more generally. Policy and practice development in supporting the child/parent relationship has primarily focused on mothers, with the consequential underplaying of the importance of the father/child relationship from the father's point of view as well as that of the child. Between 2015 and 2016, a national qualitative study, the first of its kind conducted in the Republic of Ireland, aimed to explore professional perspectives of those working in the Irish prison system on the extent to which the rights of children with a parent in prison are recognised and protected during prison visits. A small number of family members were interviewed to give some insight into the experiences of children and families. Thus, the findings of this study as they relate to the child's right to contact specifically will be presented and considered. This article adopts a children's rights framework to consider the challenges involved in realising the rights of a child when their father is in prison. Furthermore, by benchmarking current Irish practices against international and regional standards as far as child/father visits are concerned, it seeks to provide a snapshot of the extent to which the rights of children with a parent in prison are protected in the Republic of Ireland.

Introduction

In Ireland, the development of children's rights has been guided by minimum international children's rights standards as set out under the United Nations Convention on the Rights of the Child 1989 (CRC). While Irish domestic law concerning children's rights has been slow in terms of its initial development since ratification of the CRC in 1992, recent years have witnessed significant developments. These include: the appointment of a Senior Minister for Children (2011); the incorporation of some rights of children into the highest source of Irish domestic law under Article 42A of Bunreacht na hÉireann

(1937); the appointment of an Ombudsman for Children (2003) as well as the enactment of a raft of domestic legislation in the field of child law and child protection. However, while progress in the field of children's rights has been positive, children with a parent in prison have not featured in any of these developments.

Despite an absence of central government initiatives in this regard, there have been some positive moves made by the Irish Prison Service (IPS) which are primarily designed to enhance the visiting experiences of children and families. Such changes have principally been focused on improving visiting room conditions and the piloting of a parenting programme (Family Imprisonment Group, 2014); changes which, unsurprisingly, are centred around the prisoner. Yet children, in exercising their rights to see their parents, must come inside the prison walls, an experience which can often be a negative one. A failure by the prison authorities to view such visits through the lens of a child, or indeed, even being cognisant of the need to protect the human rights of children in this context, makes it impossible to adopt a child-sensitive approach to visits and potentially exposes children to damage in the long term (Tewksbury & Demichele, 2005). This is clearly at odds with the legal responsibility of the state internationally and domestically to be proactive in terms of protecting the wellbeing of all children, irrespective of who their parents are and where they reside. In the absence of such basic protections, children with a parent in prison are at risk in the short, medium and long term and the state has failed them.

It is significant therefore that the most recent policy framework on the rights of children and young people in Ireland—*Better Outcomes, Brighter Futures*—has, for the first time, given a specific State commitment to "ensure adequate access by children to an imprisoned parent, in a child-friendly setting" (Department of Children and Youth Affairs, 2014, para. 3.22). The existence of this limited commitment is of fundamental importance since it demonstrates an awareness on the part of the state of the existence of this group of children, and sets in stone a policy commitment to protect what is in fact a right of the child to have access to a parent where they have been separated from that parent as a result of a court decision.

It is in light of the latter policy commitment, that this article explores why the recognition of children's rights in the context of paternal imprisonment is fundamentally important not only in terms of protecting the international human rights of children but also in relation to supporting much needed cultural change and reform in the prison context. Moreover, existing literature concerning the role of fathers[1] in terms of parenting while in prison will be re-examined through adopting a children's rights lens, with a particular focus on children maintaining contact with their imprisoned fathers. The findings of a qualitative research project conducted in Irish prisons in 2015–2016 which sought to examine prison visits from a children's rights perspective will be considered, shining a spotlight on the existing challenges inherent in a system, the principal focus of which has traditionally been on the prisoner and prison security.

Why focus on children's rights in the context of parental incarceration?

Studies from disciplines such as psychology, sociology and criminology have focussed on the importance of maintaining family relationships once a father has been incarcerated and the barriers which can make this challenging (Brooks-Gordon & Bainham, 2004; Dyer, 2005; Jardine, 2017). While imprisonment in practice can produce a dormant period for some men in terms of fatherhood (Arditti, Smock, & Parkman, 2005), there are dangers to assuming all fathers experience imprisonment in the same way (Muth & Walker, 2013).

Despite the apparent challenges in sustaining parenting roles from inside prison, it is well accepted that there are many benefits associated with maintaining family relationships not only for the family members including children, on the outside, but also for the prisoner and the prison authorities. Fathers, in maintaining and strengthening relationships with their children while in prison, are less likely to reoffend (McCrudden, Braiden, Sloan, McCormack, & Treacy, 2014, p. 303). For the mothers on the outside, the involvement of fathers in the upbringing of their children lends itself to reduced maternal distress (Harmon & Perry, 2011). While for children, evidence suggests they can experience improved cognitive skills and behaviour (Black, Dubowitz, & Starr, 1999) as well as more responsible sexual behaviour in teenagers (Dittus, Jaccard, & Gordon, 1997).

Paternal incarceration is proven to potentially have significant and damaging consequences for the socioemotional wellbeing of children (Geller, Garfinkel, Cooper, & Mincy, 2009). The well known and respected Adverse Childhood Experiences Study carried out in the US in 1998 (Centers for Disease Control and Prevention, 2016) identified the incarceration of a family member as a risk factor for children for adult chronic disease risk behaviours (Gjelsvik, Dumont, & Nunn, 2013; Gjelsvik, Dumont, Nunn, & Rosen, 2014). The risk of childhood trauma at home or in their communities where there is the added possibility of neglect, maltreatment or violence is also increased (Arditti, 2012, p. 192). While there is also evidence to suggest that the potential effects of paternal imprisonment are higher where a child has lived with their father prior to his incarceration, it is recognised that the child who has a non-resident father is also at increased risk of family hardship in addition to being separated from a parent (Geller et al., 2009, p. 49). While some of these studies may appear dated, a more recent large-scale project involving over 1,500 children, care-givers, imprisoned parents and stakeholders across four countries (Germany, Romania, Sweden, UK) confirms many of these long-standing findings. Indeed, the final report of the well-recognised COPING Project provides rigorous and reliable data firmly rooted in science (Jones & Winaina-Wozna, 2012).

A children's rights framework to support contact with incarcerated parents

While the CRC recognises and protects the rights of all children without discrimination, certain minority groups of children have traditionally been deemed worthy of additional protection. For example, the drafters of the CRC in the 1980s included additional CRC protection for vulnerable groups such as child refugees (Art. 22), and children in conflict with the law (Arts. 37 and 40). However, during this time, little consideration was given to the rights of children with a parent in prison and, as a result, they are not specifically mentioned in the CRC.

While children with a parent in prison are theoretically entitled to the same human rights protections as any other child under the CRC, there are practical challenges for this group of children in terms of accessing these rights. At both policy and practice levels, there is a lack of systematic and targeted recognition of these children as a group in need of additional protection. The reasons for this are varied—in part they tend to be an "invisible" group, many of these children claim that they are treated as if they are guilty by association (Scharff-Smith & Gampell, 2011), which in turn can lead to both stigmatisation and marginalisation (Jones & Winaina-Wozna, 2012). In circumstances where the needs of these children are acknowledged by the state in some way, further challenges arise when a one-size-fits-all approach is generally adopted with the group being classified as either traumatised and/or likely to end up in conflict with the law themselves. While these children do have challenges in life as a result of separation from their parent in prison, there is an inherent danger of pathologising them (Knudsen, 2016).

While these children are entitled to the protection of all CRC provisions, some provisions are particularly instructive. For example, Article 3 CRC requires that where any actions taken by the state affect a child including the incarceration of a parent, the best interests of that child must be considered. Under Article 6, all children have a right to healthy development; the literature reviewed above shows parental imprisonment has the potential to negatively impact on the development of a child (Abramowicz, 2012, p. 231). Child visits can therefore be crucial under this provision; according to Poehlmann et al., " … parent-child contact during parental incarceration is a multifaceted issue that may have significant effects on children's development, caregivers' well-being, and incarcerated parents' stress, mental health, and possibly recidivism" (2010, p. 22). For children with a parent in prison, the development of secure attachments therefore involve caregiving interactions both within the home (Poehlmann et al., 2008) as well as an ongoing relationship with the parent in prison (Poehlmann, 2005). As acknowledged by Kuzucu: "Empirical evidence suggests that fathers affect their children's social, emotional and intellectual development" (Kuzucu, 2011).

The right of a child to both express their views and have such views respected in all matters affecting them (Art. 12 CRC), is one of the most empowering provisions of the CRC. In order to exercise this right effectively, children should have access to information concerning the circumstances of their parent in prison and what the right of access to that parent involves (Arts. 13 & 17 CRC). Moreover, Article 12 provides the means through which children can have their voices heard where such contact does not take place, irrespective of the reasons for this. As Liefaard highlights, while prisoners are provided with a complaint mechanism regarding their detention, "these mechanisms are not meant for children of prisoners, let alone are they child-friendly" (2015, p. 14).

International guidance?

Detailed consideration by the UN Committee on the Rights of the Child first focused on the rights of children of prisoners in 2011 during a day of general discussion on the issue. The Committee highlighted that children with a parent in prison have a right "to maintain personal relations and direct contact with both parents on a regular basis, except if it is contrary to the child's best interests" in accordance with Article 9(3) CRC (para. 35). Children have a right to visit their parent and any visits that take place must be respectful of the child's dignity and right to privacy (para. 38). The Committee also highlighted the importance of visits taking place in a child friendly environment, including by allowing visits at times that do not negatively interfere with other elements of the child's life, such as schooling, and for durations conducive to building or maintaining strong relationships. Consideration should also be made to permitting visits to take place outside the detention facility, with a view to facilitating necessary emotional bonding between the child and the incarcerated parent(s) in a child-friendly environment. (para 40)

In considering what effective child visits should look like, Poehlmann et al. underscore the importance of developing a child-sensitive approach where children are adequately prepared in accordance with their age and understanding for the visit in advance. Such preparations would include " ... providing details about what the child might see and hear at each step of the visit, informing the child of institutional rules or procedures that need to be followed, and discussing potential emotional reactions that might occur" (2010, p. 21). Furthermore, information should be given in a supportive manner where the child's questions are answered simply and honestly. Indeed, it has been established that distorted communication about a parent's incarceration leads to feelings of insecurity in young children (Poehlmann, 2005).

National law: children's rights, state responsibilities and child wellbeing

Despite the fact that in Ireland there has been a gradual shift towards ensuring that children's rights are respected in all aspects of society, the importance of adopting such a rights-based approach concerning child visits with a parent in prison has yet to become an issue of importance for the government. Arguably, this is due to a number of reasons but critically one of the main reasons is the failure of the State to see this as a child wellbeing issue. As discussed above, there are a litany of rights belonging to children which require protection, even more so when a parent is imprisoned. Where the state has made a decision which results in the separation of a parent and a child, it ultimately has a responsibility to ensure that the parent/child relationship is maintained as far as possible, where it is in the best interests of the child. It is clear that the ability of a father to parent from inside prison is severely restricted and so, as a result, it is the responsibilty of the State to facilitate contact and to promote a father/child relationship as far as is possible.

Signficantly, to date, it has been the Irish Prison Service (IPS) that has spearheaded an initiative aimed at facilitating and strengthening the father/child relationship in Irish prisons. This move to strengthen family engagement by the IPS was arguably prompted by the publication in 2012 of a report by Ireland's prison reform NGO—the Irish Penal Reform Trust (IPRT). The *Picking up the Pieces* report examined the rights and needs of families affected by imprisonment highlighting practical problems which deterred carers from taking children to visit their incarcerated parent in the Irish system. These included poor visiting conditions and frightening security measures (Martyn, 2012, pp. 31–39). In response, the IPS established a Families and Imprisonment Group (FIG). FIG was tasked with addressing some of the issues raised by the IPRT, particularly those concerning visiting conditions. The result has been the development of an IPS strategy which includes the adoption of a formal visiting policy aimed at promoting "visits, and family visits in particular, as a core element in rehabilitation" (FIG, 2014). This welcome move to formalise a family visits policy was developed across five key "pillars": (1) communications; (2) improved visiting facilities; (3) staff support and training; (4) the development of family-related courses and programmes and; (5) community follow-up and partnership with community services. Disappointingly, children are not directly included in any of these pillars. Indeed, unsurprisingly, much of the IPS developments are focused on internal actions that can support improved prison visits—physical spaces, staff training, improved communication. However, as argued below, the lack of direct engagement with the rights of children in this context is problematic in ensuring that the IPS effectively meets its children's rights obligations.

Investigating the child's right to contact with a parent in an Irish prison

Ireland has 12 prisons and places of detention; 10 are closed and two are open prisons. Prison visits operate under the Irish Prison Rules providing sentenced prisoners with one visit a week of 30 minutes in duration. However, a degree of flexibility operates within this system. Flexibility is important in facilitating improved visiting conditions, yet it can be operated inconsistently. O'Malley et al. found that women prisoners may get "outings" with their children or, a "welfare visit" may be facilitated in the community where children cannot attend the prison (2016). While positive practice of this type provides important contact particularly for children who are in care, the same degree of flexibility is not generally extended to fathers who may have similar access problems. In addition, gatekeeping by mothers and other family members on the outside can also result in restrictions being imposed on the level of contact, if any, between father and child (Rosenberg, 2009). The current study, which forms the principal focus for the remainder of this article, sought to examine the extent to which prison visiting arrangements with incarcerated fathers in Ireland conform to minimum children's rights standards set out under international law.

Methodology

Following a desktop study of research concerning the impact of parental imprisonment on children as well as a thorough search of existing Irish research in this field, it was clear that there was a dearth of research specifically examining the extent to which the rights of children to contact with a father in prison are recognised and protected in Ireland. Some key pieces of research exist which explore the recognition and protection of children's rights in the context of parental imprisonment (Lagoutte, 2016; Scharff-Smith, 2014); however, these are international in nature.

Thus, this article draws on data from qualitative research, funded by the Irish Research Council, which examined the extent to which prison visits for children with a father in prison in Ireland conform with the state's international, regional and national legal and children's rights obligations. The project was a national study which took place between 2015 and 2016 in collaboration with relevant support organisations. It was the first study of its kind to be carried out on Irish prison visits, focussing on three prison sites in Ireland.[2]

Location

For the purposes of this study, the focus was on closed prisons, one of which was a maximum-security prison and two were medium-security prisons. The maximum-security prison was chosen on the basis of location as well as with a view to providing a broader context to the Irish closed prisons for long-term prisoners. The two medium-security prisons, while also chosen on the basis of ensuring an even geographical distribution, were of particular interest as both sites were undergoing significant changes which required staff to adjust existing practices. Indeed, one prison was chosen as the location to pilot a project aimed at supporting parenting/family visits. The other was transitioning from a harsh prison environment to a modern prison approach.

The participants

The study aimed to reflect a range of views of those working in or with, the prison sector in order to examine their understanding of children's rights and the importance and operation of child-friendly visits in the Irish Prison system. In addition, by tapping into the experiences of a small number of family members, the hope was to gain an insight into how visiting conditions are experienced in practice by children and families. It is acknowledged that the numbers of participants were small; however, the views presented were largely consistent.

Table 1 demonstrates the participants who were interviewed. Access to prison staff was facilitated by the Prison Governors while access to family members was provided by family support organisations. A purposive sample comprising prison governors, prison officers, child care workers and representatives from support organisations as well as those directly impacted upon by the imprisonment of a father, were invited to participate in the study. This was designed to ensure that the diverse perspectives on parental imprisonment were presented in a fair and balanced way. Participants were asked about their views regarding visiting arrangements for children, their understanding of children's rights in relation to child visits, and the relevant policy framework.

Ethics and permissions

Ethical approval was sought both from the researchers' academic institution and the Irish prison service. Following this, permission was sought from the Head of the Irish Prison Service for the purposes of contacting the relevant Governors. Once permission was secured, the prison governors were invited for interview and each prison then provided staff who volunteered to be interviewed. No one refused to be interviewed. All participants were given an information sheet detailing the nature and scope of the study, they were

Table 1. Study participants.

Profession/Role	Format	No of participants
Family members	Semi-structured interviews	3[a] (n = 2 + 1)
Irish Prison Service—Senior Administration	Semi-structured interviews	1
Irish Prison Service: Governors	Semi-structured interviews	4
Irish Prison Service—Prison Officers	Semi-structured interviews	2
Prison Support Staff—		
Child Care Worker	Semi-structured interviews	1
Support Organisations	Semi-structured interviews	2[b] (n = 3)

[a]There were three family members interviewed in total; two of these were a mother and daughter from the same family.
[b]Three professionals working with community support organisations were interviewed; two of these were representing one organisation.

reminded that participation was voluntary and they were asked to sign an informed consent form.

Limitations of the study

While this study sought to examine Irish prison visits through the lens of a child by adopting a children's rights framework, the researchers were aware of the fact that children below the age of 18 years were not directly involved in this phase of the research. While this limited the parameters of the research findings, the researchers will expand this research in the future to include the voices of children, when all appropriate safeguards can be put in place. In addition, it is recognised that the sample size is relatively small and therefore, the results are not reflective of the views of everyone with direct experience of the system.

Research analysis and findings: children's rights and maintaining contact with fathers in prison in Ireland

A qualitative methodology was employed for the study using semi-structured interviews as a means of data collection, with the data being analysed using thematic analysis, the latter being a well-recognised "method for identifying, analysing and reporting patterns in the data" (Braun & Clarke, 2006, p. 79). The same interview schedule was used for all interviews ensuring that the same format was employed throughout. Interview times varied with some lasting one hour, others as much as two-and-a-half hours. Each interview was recorded via dictaphone and later transcribed verbatim. Interviews were coded and themes were created using a theoretical or deductive method which was to some extent influenced by the researchers' theoretical interest in this area. While it is well accepted that the latter form of analysis lends itself to providing a less " … rich description of the data overall", it does help construct a realistic picture of aspects of the data (Braun & Clarke, 2006, p. 84). In relation to the professionals, the focus was on the participants understanding of their own actions particularly as part of the system operating around them. It was striking that the majority of professionals interviewed spoke more in the context and language of child protection rather than children's rights. This paternalistic approach was not surprising given the fact that child protection and understanding thereof is embedded in practices and procedures and is buttressed by the existence of child protection legislation. Moreover, there is no children's rights-based training currently available for prison professionals. It is important to point out that the views highlighted below were chosen due to their representativeness of those expressed by professionals working within the system more generally. Where views were expressed that differed from the norm, these are identified as such.

Emerging themes

As a result of the coding process, themes emerged from the study in relation to a number of areas. Given the focus of this piece, just four of these will be discussed relating specifically to the child's right to maintain contact with a parent (Art. 9 CRC). A child's contact with his or her father must be meaningful in the sense that the conditions before the visit takes place and thereafter must be children's rights-compliant. Further, contact should be a right protected for all children with a father in prison irrespective of where they live or prison disciplinary regimes.

Unsurprisingly, perceptions varied amongst the participants with the focus of prison staff being primarily that of prison security, while family members tended to talk about their experience of visitation within the prison and the quality of their experiences. Interestingly, from a children's rights perspective, one family member had a very clear view on where children fit in terms of the priorities of the prison:

> I think children are overlooked by the prison services. I know there are other agencies lobbying for children's rights but I just feel that they are not important really in the Prison Service's eyes, they are just about the prisoner and the security and managing that whereas children really don't come into their minds at all I don't think. (Family member 1, County B)

Understandings of children's rights within the prison context

While prison personnel were aware of the fact that they have some responsibility towards children visiting their father in prison, this appeared to be mainly from a child protection point of view, rather than a children's rights perspective.

> [W]e are very much focused on child protection here; it's around child protection rather than about development. ... I don't think society has gone on to the whole development of a child thing yet ... . We've got the child protection, which took us 100 years to get to, and now we're looking at protecting the child first and we haven't gone on to children's rights yet. And it's an awareness that some people have but I don't think we've *even* got there. (Governor 1, Prison A) [own emphasis added]

Similarly, even when talking about future developments and demonstrating awareness of the potential challenges, child protection remained a key priority, without any consideration of the broader children's rights framework. One Governor interviewee highlighted the cultural challenge of "subverting" the security dynamic to allow for a more relaxed approach, being placed alongside:

> ... challenging the family and the prisoner around their responsibility on the visit. I think they are the critical things, and also I understand we need to be aware of any potential issues around child protection in allowing you know. I mean all of the legislation says that we should encourage family contact where it's not detrimental to the child. So we need to have a mechanism of picking up those bits as well, so that we don't, you know so you must visit your child ... (Governor 1, Prison B)

At the heart of the prison approach was the idea that the IPS was just beginning a process of change, "There's a long journey to go and we're just about starting that journey really" (Senior Prison Official). However, the danger here is that that journey paradigm may result in the justification of extremely slow progress which prevents the IPS from meeting its obligations towards children. Placed alongside one of the most poignant representations of children's rights from a family member when recalling how her daughter reacted to the visit system in the past, the tension is clear:

> I remember going back a couple of years ago when her father was in prison she used to always say to me "that it's my right to have physical contact with my father". I can remember her saying that years ago. ... I remember she used to say ... "Well my rights were took away

and I didn't do any crime", she was still being punished which is wrong like, that the rights of the child should be the fact that they can have physical and emotional contact with their parents in prison, like a hug won't kill anyone like and at least it keeps that child nourished and knowing that they're loved or … like I'd hate to be in prison and the fact that my little girl or my others couldn't come up and hug me. (Family member 1, County A)

Unfortunately, there was little or no awareness of the relevance or applicability of children's rights within the context of prison visits amongst prison staff at all levels, despite the obligation on the government under Article 42 CRC to publicise the rights of children within the domestic sphere: "we haven't stepped over into thinking about children's rights at any stage" (Governor 1, Prison A). Similarly, one professional working in another prison admitted: "I don't know what the children's rights are so I can't implement a policy when I don't know what their rights are" (Prison Officer 1, Prison C). Indeed, when asked about how children's rights could be better understood in the prison context, "Just information and training" (Governor 1, Prison B) was the response of one prison governor.

Yet the practical experience of family members upon entering the prison from a human rights point of view was abundantly apparent from one participant: "I suppose I feel that as soon as they [children of prisoners] enter the gate of the prison they actually lose all their rights as well, as well as you as a human being lose your rights" (Family member 1, County B).

Experiences of visiting from a children's rights perspective

The experiences of children visiting a parent in prison in Ireland tend to vary to a large degree. This is owing to a number of factors including the type of prison a parent is held in, the level of security of the prison, and the prison culture. Indeed, as acknowledged by one Prison Governor, "We're independent serfdoms, call it what you like" (Prison Governor 1, County B). Yet, all children have a right to be treated equally (Art. 2 CRC) in terms of maintaining contact with their parent in prison (Art. 9 CRC).

In certain circumstances, the nature and extent of contact, when it occurs, is dictated by the behaviour of the father in prison. In particular, the enhanced visits regime in Ireland is designed to encourage better behaviour on the part of the prisoners. However, in reality, the regime directly impacts on a child's right to access their father in prison in the short term; while in the long term it will impact on the father/child relationship and will potentially affect the child's long-term development.

[I]f you're on enhanced … I do get the whole idea of enhanced visits but I still think that it's unfair for children that it's only if Daddy is good that they'll get to touch him. I think it should be full contact at all times, obviously within reason. I know there are times if there are contraband being brought in that they will have to have screen visits and stuff but I personally don't agree with that whole approach, that if you're good and behave and follow everything that you're supposed to in prison then you can touch your children and you can kiss them and hug them but if you're bad you can't. So I think it's punishing the children as opposed to punishing the prisoner. (Family member 1, County B)

For the most part, standard visits in a closed prison setting are perceived by family members as being poor: "They're not a bit child-friendly" (Family member 1, County A).

There was some evidence of positive practice and a strong awareness of the need to promote the rights of children when they are visiting their father in prison. This was the exception as opposed to the norm however. According to one visiting room support worker:

> [I]t's important for ... the childcare workers to be here for the children, to listen to them and what they have to say where sometimes they just get dragged along in the whole process and it is important for them to have a voice .... (Prison Visiting room worker, County C)

The need to recognise that formal visits are inadequate to support meaningful child/parent contact is well established. Clarke et al found that " ... men's accounts ... showed the tensions of attempting to condense family interaction into intense, spatially constrained visits and telephone time slots" (Clarke et al., 2005). Acknowledging this reality, one interviewee highlighted the need to develop an "understanding of the wants and needs of the family unit" that goes beyond the mere physical space of visits:

> [I]t's not just okay you have the room right .... You know you are trying to have a normal family interaction of an evening around homework or around whatever is going on. And again, I think those that visit with the use of our child officer and all the rest could become very focused on what the family needs to achieve in that time you know. So ... the barrier is your imagination, in terms of you know, within the parameters of the security piece .... (Governor 1, Prison B)

Visiting can therefore be enhanced through a variety of enhanced, child-centred, interventions: homework clubs, the organisation of parent-teacher meetings and family activity visits.

Barriers to supporting the parent/child relationship and a child's right to meaningful contact

In reality, there were a number of barriers identified to ensuring the child has a meaningful relationship with their father in prison and vice versa, including obstacles of an attitudinal as well as a physical nature. In particular, negative attitudes towards a father's ability to parent were demonstrated by prison staff. A senior IPS interviewee expressed some frustration with the engagement of parents in their children's lives in the context of imprisonment, despite being committed to supporting family relationships:

> I think sometimes we leave the adults off the hook a bit in terms of their responsibility for the child and, like, their responsibility for understanding where the child is, what age they are, what class they're in, what type of age-appropriate material they should be looking at, they should be dealing with. I mean they have to take ... responsibility for their children, not just us. (Senior IPS official)

The idea of fathers being responsible for their own role was a common theme throughout the interviews. However, this concern was not placed within a consistent and purposeful examination of the real opportunities for fathers to do anything other than a visit and have phone calls with their child. One Governor noted that this was not just about "parenting" but related to wider capacity barriers that prisoners experience:

> [I]t's about the prisoners' kind of manning up, for want of a better word, to what their issues are. Because if a person can't read and write, they're going to be no good to their children or their homework. So it's a matter of normalising things. (Governor 1, Prison A)

The juxtaposition in this approach—the need to "man up" on the one hand and the actual capacity of some incarcerated parents—illustrates the tensions in viewing parenting as a one-dimensional rather than multi-dimensional aspect of prisoners' lives.

One prison officer went so far as to say that fathers had little interest in their children:

> [Y]ou have the prisoners that it's like they don't really care, that they just want to get the visit over and done with, they're more interested in their girlfriend than their child … . (Prison Officer, County C)

By comparison, family members highlighted the reality for the parent in prison:

> Essentially, it's like as if when a man goes to prison he loses his status as a father. Nobody cares. You are a prisoner now and you're not a father and it doesn't matter which is wrong … … .they lose their status and then when they come out that's extremely hard to build back up again. They lose their identity as a parent inside and then on release that's quite difficult to gain back again. (Partner 1, County B)

Even the physical structure of the normal visiting rooms or boxes are not necessarily suitable for ensuring quality visits between children and their fathers. One family member explained the reality from a father's point of view:

> Do you know like I mean if the child is having problems at school and things like this and when you go in you want the father to be able to play a part, a role in the child's life, to be able to say like "Well look I know what happened to you at school", this and that, but it can't be done. If there was a bit more space in the visiting box that he could sit down and talk to the child or she could sit down and talk to the child about whatever was going on in their life, that there is a need for more space, just so many feet between each prisoner, because one prisoner can go back and tell everyone else on the landing what's been happening on his visit, do you know, so. (Family Member 1, County A)

Opportunities for moving forward

Without fixing child-centred actions formally into policy, such interventions are rarely if ever embedded into prison practice, both at the local and national level. One Governor expressed frustration at this situation:

> anything that we've achieved here is because I'm here. And that shouldn't be the way. It shouldn't depend on me. I always say that about the job. It shouldn't be about … [Individual personalities and their own ethos]. … Because when I walk away from here, that should continue. It shouldn't roll back and say, well, look, thank god that lunatic's gone, because now we can get it back to a secure prison and put the eggshell paint back on the walls. (Governor 1, County C)

Some participants highlighted areas that could be improved upon in the future. For example, the partner of a father in prison highlighted what she considered basic requirements for a meaningful visit for her child:

> I think they need privacy. I think they need to be able to have physical contact with their family member. For older kids, they need to have that space to discuss things that are troubling them. I think younger kids should be allowed to bring in some kind of a toy or … a comfort blanket. [T]hings like that to make them feel secure because it's not a very nice place. They could be made more child friendly, colourful paintings on the wall or if they do colour in pictures in the waiting room to be allowed to bring them in with them

because it's … an achievement, they don't get to show their father their achievements really. So, little things like that I think would be good … they need to have proper quality time when they are on visits not all crammed into the one tiny room fighting for conversation. (Family member 1, County B)

The need for a dedicated officer in the prison who would support meaningful visits from a children's rights perspective was identified by one family member:

if there was an officer specific for families, so like a family liaison officer … , … that would be good because they have a link, the families have a link to the prison then and the prisoner also has a link to the family I think also that person could be responsible for enforcing children's rights within prisons but that's a long way off. (Family member 1, County B)

A visiting room support worker highlighted what she considered important in terms of best practice from a children's rights point of view:

Best practice in this area is to be open to everybody and all the issues coming in and to understand from a parent's point of view coming here but to be here for the children, that you are here for them, that when they come in they can have a good time here. (Prison Visiting room worker, County C)

Conclusion: developing a children's rights approach to prison visits

This article has sought to examine the extent to which the rights of children with a parent in prison are respected in the context of child prison visits in the Republic of Ireland. As demonstrated by the findings, there is a clear dissonance between how the rights of this group of innocent children should be protected in theory under the CRC and how that compares with their practical experiences of prison visits in the Irish context. Despite the absence of structured guidance from the UN Committee on the Rights of the Child through the form of a general comment in this area, existing CRC provisions require the development and implementation of a child-sensitive approach to child visits that is consistently and systematically applied across the Irish prison estate. In addition, such an approach should not be linked to the good behaviour of prisoners. All children of prisoners are entitled to child-sensitive visiting arrangements; except where there is evidence that such visits are not in the child's bests interests. It is therefore recommended that all children be provided with "enhanced" family visits which focus on visiting arrangements whereby they can interact with their imprisoned parent in a constructive way. This should include the adoption of homework clubs in all prisons and opportunities for prisoners to eat and play with their children in a relaxed environment.

It is argued that a children's rights-based approach should be used in the development of any ongoing prison training, as well as in the future development of prison policies which affect children as required under international law. More predominantly, a children's rights approach is one which, on a practical level, serves to benefit everyone affected when a father is incarcerated including the child, the parents, society and the prison. Such an approach would allow for a non-discriminatory approach where children of both mothers and fathers would be offered gender-appropriate supports and contact with their parent in custody. This does not require universal forms of intervention, since families affected by parental imprisonment are not a homogenous group. Indeed, there is a need to recognise that there may be unique needs of all concerned.

A shift in perspective is proposed—moving the focus from what may be a discriminatory and problematic approach to adopting a more nuanced and variable range of interventions that can support and develop child/father interactions. Such interventions should be tailored to the needs of individual families in a way that avoids pathologising children and their fathers within the system. Under the current FIG programme, there is evidence of a commitment to seeking change. However, to date, the journey towards meeting the rights of children visiting their parent in prison has been slow and modest. It is necessary for the State and by extension, the IPS, to recognise that children's rights are not a luxury, but a responsibility imposed by international law. The professionals working within the prison system can provide the space and opportunity to support children and their parents to maintain and develop strong relationships that are beneficial to all. They are gatekeepers to this relationship, in the same way that parents and carers outside the prison are.

Notes

1. While much research exists concerning maternal imprisonment and its impact on children and young people, the focus of this article is on fathers only.
2. While three sites formed the focus, four prisons formed the focus of this study.

Disclosure statement

No potential conflict of interest was reported by the authors.

Funding

This work was supported by Irish Research Council for the Humanities and Social Sciences: [Grant Number New Foundations Award 2014–15].

References

Abramowicz, S. (2012). A family law perspective on parental incarceration. *Family Court Review, 50* (2), 228–240.

Arditti, J. (2012). Child trauma within the context of parental incarceration: A family process perspective. *Journal of Family Theory & Review, 4*(September), 181–219.

Arditti, J., Smock, S. A., & Parkman, T. S. (2005). "It's been hard to be a father": A qualitative exploration of incarcerated fatherhood. *Fathering: A Journal of Theory, Research, and Practice About Men as Fathers, 3*(3), 267–288.

Black, M. M., Dubowitz, H., & Starr, R. H., Jr. (1999). African American fathers in low income, urban families: Development, behavior, and home environment of their Three-Year-Old children. *Child Development, 70*(4), 967–978.

Braun, V., & Clarke, V. (2006). Using thematic analysis in psychology. *Qualitative Research in Psychology, 3,* 77–101.

Brooks-Gordon, B., & Bainham, A. (2004). Prisoners' families and the regulation of contact. *Journal of Social Welfare and Family Law, 26*(3), 263–280.

Bunreacht na hÉireann (Constitution of Ireland). (1937). Article 42A.

Centers for Disease Control and Prevention. (2016). *Violence prevention.* [Online] Retrieved from https://www.cdc.gov/violenceprevention/acestudy/about_ace.html

Clarke, L., O'Brien, M., Day, R. D., Godwin, H., Connolly, J., Hemmings, J., & Van Leeson, T. (2005). Fathering behind bars in English prisons: Imprisoned fathers' identity and contact with their children. *Fathering: A Journal of Theory, Research, and Practice About Men as Fathers, 3*(3), 221–241.

Committee on the Rights of the Child. (2011). *Report and recommendations of the Day of general discussion on "children of incarcerated parents".* Geneva: United Nations.

Department of Children and Youth Affairs. (2014). *Better outcomes, brighter futures: The national policy framework for children and young people 2014–2020.* Dublin: Author.

Dittus, P. J., Jaccard, J., & Gordon, V. V. (1997). The impact of African American fathers on adolescent sexual behavior. *Journal of Youth and Adolescence, 26*(4), 445–465.

Dyer, J. (2005). Prison, fathers, and identity: A theory of how incarceration affects men's paternal identity. *Fathering: A Journal of Theory, Research, and Practice About Men as Fathers, 3*(3), 201–219.

Families and Imprisonment Group. (2014). *Report to director general.* Irish Prison Service.

Geller, A., Garfinkel, I., Cooper, C., & Mincy, R. (2009). Parental incarceration and child well-being: Implications for urban families. *Social Science Quarterly, 90,* 1186–1202.

Gjelsvik, A., Dumont, D., & Nunn, A. (2013, May). Incarceration of a household member and Hispanic health disparities: Childhood exposure and adult chronic disease risk behaviors. *Preventing Chronic Disease, 10*(10), 69.

Gjelsvik, A., Dumont, D., Nunn, A., & Rosen, D. (2014, August). Adverse childhood events: Incarceration of household members and health-related quality of life in adulthood. *Journal of Health Care for the Poor and Underserved, 25*(3), 1169–1182.

Harmon, D., & Perry, A. R. (2011). Fathers' unaccounted contributions: Parental involvement and maternal stress. *Families in Society, 92,* 176–182.

Jardine, C. (2017). Constructing and maintaining family in the context of imprisonment. *British Journal of Criminology, 58,* 114–131.

Jones, A., & Winaina-Wozna, A. (2012). *COPING: Children of prisoners, interventions and mitigations to strengthen mental health.* European Commission.

Knudsen, E. M. (2016). Avoiding the pathologizing of children of prisoners. *Probation Journal, 63* (3), 362–370.

Kuzucu, Y. (2011). The changing role of fathers and its impact on child development. *Turkish Psychological Counseling and Guidance Journal, 4*(35), 79–91.

Lagoutte, S. (2016). The right to respect for family life of children of imprisoned parents. *The International Journal of Children's Rights, 24,* 204–230.

Liefaard, T. (2015). Rights of children of incarcerated parents: Towards more procedural safeguards. *European Journal of Parental Imprisonment, 1*(Spring), 13–15.

Martyn, M. (2012). *"Picking up the pieces": The rights and needs of children and families affected by parental imprisonment.* Dublin: IPRT.

McCrudden, E., Braiden, H. J., Sloan, D., McCormack, P., & Treacy, A. (2014). Stealing the smile from my child's face: A preliminary evaluation of the "being a dad" programme in a Northern Ireland prison. *Child Care in Practice, 20*(3), 301–312.

Muth, W., & Walker, G. (2013). Looking up: The temporal horizons of a father in prison. *Fathering: A Journal of Theory, Research, and Practice About Men as Fathers, 11*(3), 292–305.

O'Malley, S., & Devaney, C. (2016). Maintaining the mother–child relationship within the Irish prison system: The practitioner perspective. *Child Care in Practice, 22*, 20–34.

Poehlmann, J. (2005). Representations of attachment relationships in children of incarcerated mothers. *Child Development, 76*, 679–696.

Poehlmann, J., Dallaire, D., Booker Loper, A., & Shear, L. D. (2010). Children's contact with their incarcerated parents: Research findings and recommendations. *American Psychology, September, 65*(6), 575–598.

Poehlmann, J., Park, J., Bouffiou, L., Abrahams, J., Shlafer, R., & Hahn, E. (2008). Representations of family relationships in children living with custodial grandparents. *Attachment and Human Development, 10*, 165–188.

Rosenberg, J. (2009). *Children need dads too: Children with fathers in prison.* Geneva: Quaker United National Office.

Scharff-Smith, P. (2014). Children of imprisoned parents in Scandinavia: Their problems, treatment and the role of Scandinavian penal culture. *Law in Context, 32*, 147–168.

Scharff-Smith, P., & Gampell, L. (2011). *Children of imprisoned parents.* Copenhagen: Danish Institute for Human Rights.

Tewksbury, R., & Demichele, M. (2005). Going to prison: A prison visitation program. *The Prison Journal, 85*(3), 292–310.

Recruiting, Retaining and Engaging Men in Social Interventions: Lessons for Implementation Focusing on a Prison-based Parenting Intervention for Young Incarcerated Fathers

Katie Buston

ABSTRACT

Recruiting, retaining and engaging men in social interventions can be challenging. The focus of this paper is the successful implementation of a parenting programme for incarcerated fathers, delivered in a Young Offender Institution (YOI) in Scotland. Reasons for high levels of recruitment, retention and engagement are explored, with barriers identified. A qualitative design was employed using ethnographic approaches including participant observation of the programme, informal interactions, and formal interviews with programme participants, the facilitators and others involved in managing the programme. Framework analysis was conducted on the integrated data set. The prison as the setting for programme delivery was both an opportunity and a challenge. It enabled easy access to participants and required low levels of effort on their part to attend. The creation of a nurturing and safe environment within the prison classroom facilitated engagement: relationships between the facilitators and participants, and between the participants themselves were key to understanding high levels of retention and engagement. The most fundamental challenge to high engagement levels arose from clashes in embedded institutional ways of working, between the host institution and the organisation experienced in delivering such intervention work. This threatened to compromise trust between the participants and the facilitators. Whilst adding specifically to the very sparse literature on reaching incarcerated young fathers and engaging them in parenting work, the findings have transferability to other under-researched areas: the implementation of social interventions generally in the prison setting, and engaging marginalised fathers in parenting/family work in community settings. The paper highlights ways of overcoming some of the challenges faced.

Introduction

Interventions for fathers are a recent growth area in family services; effectively representing fathers is a policy priority. There is now little doubt that fathers matter for the welfare of children and adults (Flouri & Buchanan, 2002, 2003, 2004; Flouri, Buchanan, & Bream, 2002; Kim, Kang, Yee, Shim, & Chung, 2016; Kroll, Carson, Redshaw, & Quigley, 2016). Programmes that potentially increase fathers' involvement with their children are seen as an important complement to those that target mothers (Lundahl, Tollefson, Risser, & Lovejoy, 2008; Scourfield, Yi Cheung, & Macdonald, 2014). While there is established evidence that parenting interventions generally can be effective, the evidence base for parenting interventions which target fathers is much less developed and definitive. Studies which have been conducted, however, suggest that such parenting interventions may be effective in improving fathers' involvement with their children (Bronte-Tinkew et al., 2008; Cowan, Cowan, Pruett, Pruett, & Wong, 2009; Magill-Evans, Harrison, Rempel, & Slater, 2006; Philip & O'Brien, 2012; Smith, Duggan, Bair-Merritt, & Cox, 2012).

Engagement in parenting interventions has been conceptualised as a sequential process, involving (a) initial take-up in response to recruitment procedures; (b) retention whereby participants return for the full course; (c) engagement with the delivery of the programme demonstrated by participation and interest (Lindsay et al., 2008; Moran, Ghate, & van der Merwe, 2004). There is some useful literature identifying the potential barriers parents face in engaging with parenting programmes, though there is little robust evidence as to "what works" (Axford, Lehtonen, Kaoukji, Tobin, & Berry, 2012; Katz, La Placa, & Hunter, 2007). The factors key to successful implementation appear to be whether parents can build up a trusting relationship with the front line service providers, and the degree to which parents feel they are in control of the help they are receiving.

Most studies around engagement in this area have focused on mothers (Panter-Brick et al., 2014). There is evidence that parenting programmes, and mainstream family services generally, fail to engage fathers (Maxwell, Scourfield, Featherstone, Holland, & Tolman, 2012; Scourfield et al., 2014). Bayley, Wallace, and Choudhry (2009) found that fathers tend to interpret the word "parent" as meaning mother when it is used on literature to advertise family services. Berlyn, Wise, and Soriano (2008) found that fathers were intimidated by the idea of accessing any sort of family support. In a study of young fathers' experiences of the Family Nurse Partnership, Ferguson (2016) identified that their non-engagement arose from a combination of service delivery issues and from complexities around their own vulnerabilities and prior negative experiences as service users. Feeling excluded and/or judged are common experiences for young fathers, shaping their attitude to accessing family services (Fletcher & Visser, 2008; Ross, Church, Hill, Seaman, & Roberts, 2012), and seeking or receiving help is regarded as unmasculine (O'Brien, Hunt, & Hart, 2005).

There is also some work that suggests that parents living in poverty are more likely to be stressed and depressed, and this may hinder them from accessing parenting support (Katz, Corlyon, La Placa, & Hunter, 2007). In general, parents in areas of concentrated poverty often feel they lack the skills to become more involved.

Young parents, including fathers, also tend to be disadvantaged, in a number of ways which do not facilitate straightforward access to parenting support. Men who become fathers at a young age tend to have an accumulation of risk factors: low social class, early risk behaviour including sexual activity and substance use, mental health problems, lack of social support, and low educational attainment (Barlow et al., 2011; Buston, Parkes, Thomson, Wight, & Fenton, 2012). They tend to know little about child development or effective parenting skills (Barlow et al., 2011).

Being incarcerated exacerbates disadvantage still further, with any contact the father has with his child(ren) compromised by the period of his incarceration (Kazura, 2001; Nurse, 2001). Around one in four incarcerated young offenders in the UK are estimated to be actual or expectant fathers (Macmillan, 2005). There is a clear need for parenting interventions for young offender fathers to help them fulfil their roles as fathers, given the multi-faceted nature of their disadvantage, and to improve outcomes for their children (Lundahl et al., 2008) and themselves (Barlow et al., 2011). This need has been recognised and parenting intervention work has, indeed, been delivered in Young Offender Institutions (YOIs) in the UK for around 25 years (Buston et al., 2012), but has been characterised by patchiness and non-sustainability. There are few published process evaluations of parenting programmes in prisons (Miller et al., 2014), and none that the author is aware of in relation to interventions for young incarcerated fathers. A review of family interventions more broadly in the prison environment concluded that there were problems delivering such interventions in this setting because of: limited engagement with families, high participant drop-out rates, prisoner concerns about confidentiality, practical barriers such as lack of suitable rooms, and low trust between prisoners and staff (Roberts et al., 2016).

Objectives

To contribute to filling the knowledge gap in relation to marginalised men and family interventions, and to add to the sparse literature on understanding implementation of social interventions in the prison setting, this paper reports results from a process evaluation of a prison-based parenting programme for incarcerated young fathers in a Young Offender Institution (YOI) in Scotland, UK during 2015. Recruitment, retention and engagement are the focus; facilitating and constraining factors are identified. The concluding discussion focuses on the prison as a setting for such work, highlighting specific opportunities and challenges encountered by this prison-based programme.

Methods

In early 2014 the Scottish Prison Service (SPS) tendered for a third sector organisation to develop parenting services within HMP YOI Polmont, Scotland's only YOI. At that time, and for the duration of the study, it had a capacity of just over 800 male prisoners, aged 16–21 years. Run by the SPS, strategic decisions around the institution, as is the case for all the SPS establishments, are made in conjunction with the Scottish Government. Contributing to the new vision for the prison service, which is increasingly expanding beyond protecting the public and reducing reoffending (Scottish Prison Service, 2013), the strategy for young offenders is to develop the institution as a learning environment. A key development area within this is Parenting and Families. Barnardo's Scotland, a charitable organisation which works with vulnerable children, young people and their families to transform the children's lives, won the tender to develop Parenting Services. Two Parenting Officers, Prison Officers employed by SPS, were recruited to facilitate this development and to co-deliver the core parenting intervention work.

In June 2014 Barnardo's Scotland approached the author to evaluate early implementation of the core parenting programme, with the aim that results would feed into the development of the programme and to future delivery. *Parenting Matters* (an established parenting course delivered for over 20 years, largely in Northern Ireland) was used as a foundation for the programme, adapted for the incarcerated young fathers within HMP YOI Polmont. The resultant *Being a Young Dad* programme was delivered by the Barnardo's Scotland facilitator and one of the two Parenting Officers over a full day a week for 10 consecutive weeks, with a condensed six-week version available for those men due to be released within these 10 weeks. It included information, skills and more reflectively based sessions. Sessions included: "what children need from parents", "attachment", "self-esteem", "the importance of play", "positive disciplining", "behaviour management", and "budgeting". The Parenting Officers had also recruited a Peer Mentor from the group of long-term prisoners who had attended one of the first programme deliveries. His role was to help the Parenting Officers recruit fathers for future groups, and to reiterate key learning messages as well to help with practical tasks.

The programme was voluntary and open to fathers who, in theory if not always in practice, had access to their child(ren), or who had the prospect of such access. The 10-week programme included three additional and enhanced family visits, including a final celebratory visit, incorporating an award ceremony which marked the end of the programme.

The primary aim of *Being a Young Dad* was to help young fathers understand the positive role they could play in their child's life, if they chose to do so. Key to the programme theory was the development of a positive relationship between participants and facilitators, and amongst the participants themselves. It was posited that if this could be achieved the young men would feel more relaxed and supported and would therefore engage to a greater degree, and actively participate in the programme, setting the context for behavioural change. Through the process of sharing and reflecting on their experiences it was theorised that they would realise the importance of the role of father, and this would motivate them to change, drawing on other skills taught during the course. As well as working through the formal content of sessions, the atmosphere created within the classroom session was regarded by Barnardo's Scotland as key. Informal discussion, playing board games, and generally relaxing together were essential components of the course, alongside the traditional worksheet, materials on DVD, and directed discussions. Barnardo's Scotland requested a kettle and fridge for the classroom, and the facilitator provided milk and biscuits at each session in order that the young men could help themselves to refreshments. Money was also spent on resources for the programme, including games such as Monopoly, a stock of occasion cards they could send to loved ones, a radio for background music, and bean bags for relaxation.

After receiving permission from both the SPS Research and Ethics Committee and Glasgow University's Social Science Ethics Committee (400130248), the process evaluation commenced, comprising a qualitative study, using multiple methods, of the programme implementation:

(1) Participant observation of delivery of all the parenting sessions of the programme ($n = 10$ sessions), and some of the sessions ($n = 4$ sessions) of another group who were undertaking the condensed version of the programme over six weeks. Each "session" comprised a full day, divided into a morning and an afternoon with the men returning to the halls at lunchtime. Between February and April 2015 over 100 hours was spent by the author in the parenting classroom, observing, and

participating in, the programme delivery and "hanging around" between sessions talking to the staff and the young men.

(2) Attendance at family visits ($n = 3$) in the visiting room, providing an opportunity to observe some of the young men interacting with their child(ren) and their partners, or ex-partners, during the two-hour visit period.

(3) In-depth interviews ($n = 6$) with the young men who had completed the programme and who were still in the prison six weeks after its completion. The topic guide for these interviews included exploration of their motivation for attending the course, and of their views around how they were approached to participate in it; and how they felt about the programme itself exploring aspects around their participation and engagement.

(4) An in-depth interview ($n = 1$) and numerous conversations with Barnardo's managers and other staff before, during, and after the fieldwork period.

(5) Prolonged contact with those involved in delivery during the analysis period, with occasional discussions (in person and by email) about emerging results, including in the context of continuing delivery of the programme following the period of fieldwork.

(6) Collection of copies of the end of programme reports written by one of the facilitators for each man in her case load ($n = 8$). These commented systematically on attendance, the sessions covered and the individual men's engagement with the course and with particular aspects of it.

(7) Collection of written materials about the programme and its delivery, passed on by the facilitators and those within Barnardo's Scotland who introduced the programme to HMP YOI Polmont.

For (1) and (2) and the conversations referred to in (4), detailed ethnographic fieldnotes were written on leaving the prison, aided by the notes taken during the day, often in code, as an aide memoire of the day's structure. These included notes on what was delivered, by whom and how, and who was there and to what extent did they participate and how, including who said what—formally and in conversation with the author, as well as overheard. For (3) and (4) the in-depth interviews were recorded and transcribed with participants' permission. For conversations which took place with staff outside the prison—in person, by email or on the telephone—pertinent comments were recorded in a Word file which was added to the integrated data set.

All of these data sources have been analysed in an integrated way for this paper (Saldana, 2013). Barnardo's were keen to learn how the intervention was being implemented: what was being delivered, how was it being delivered, and how were the participants receiving it (that is reacting to it, and engaging with it). The data were coded by the author, initially in a descriptive way followed by more explanatory work, in order to answer these questions. "Recruitment", "retention" and "engagement" were coding categories, and within these "nodes", facilitating and constraining factors were identified, for example "trust", "institutional practices", and "practical issues". Framework analysis was used with examples charted in order to manage and summarise the voluminous data (Gale, Heath, Cameron, Rashid, & Redwood, 2013; Ritchie & Lewis, 2003).

Where quotes from young men are presented, below, a pseudonym is used. Pseudonyms have also been used for the prison staff.

Findings

Sixteen fathers participated in the two programme deliveries observed. These included those with long-term sentences, as well as those with shorter sentences and remand prisoners. The men were aged between 17 and 21 years, and had between one and three children. Some were still in a relationship with the mother of their child(ren) but most were not. Nearly all had some current contact with their child(ren).

Recruitment

The primary way of identifying and approaching fathers within the YOI in order to recruit them was through the Parenting Officers, and the Peer Mentor, attending Induction. Induction is when new prisoners are introduced to the rules, guidelines, and processes of the prison, including how visiting works and what job opportunities exist. They talked to the new arrivals during this session, and asked them whether they were fathers, or expectant fathers. The Parenting Officers and Peer Mentor then followed up those who had identified themselves as such, checked that they were eligible to receive the core programme, and visited their cells to tell them about what the core parenting programme involved, answering any questions, and inviting them along to the first session. The Parenting Officers estimate that, since they began delivering the programme around two and a half years ago, fewer than 5% of the men they have approached in this way said that they were not interested in attending. According to the Parenting Officers most of the small number who did decline did so because of the complexity of their relationship with the mother of their child and future prospects of developing a relationship with the child because of this. A small number of men were recruited through Addictions, and other, workers telling them about the programme during one-to-one sessions where their parenting was discussed.

Retention

Nearly all of those men who attended the first session of the various deliveries of the programme that have been run to date, including all of those attending the deliveries observed for this study, went on to attend the rest of the programme. It was common, however, for individual men to miss two or three mornings or afternoons of the programme due to occurrences such as court appearances, health centre or social work appointments, or hall lockdown. For the shorter course observed, two men were liberated before the end of the course. Aside from these events beyond the control of the individual men, however, attendance was high. None of the men participating in the deliveries observed for this study intentionally missed particular mornings or afternoons because they decided not to attend; all appeared committed to the programme, none dropped out. Commitment to attending was very high.

Engagement

Furthermore, all of the men observed for this study appeared to engage with the programme on a consistent basis, though actively participating in different ways and to varying extents. Timmy, for example, was quiet, rarely contributing verbally, but was on task with most of the activities, including filling in worksheets and creating a book for his baby. Jimmy, on the other hand, verbally contributed frequently, often making jokes. He liked to "banter" with the facilitators, with this sometimes crossing the line into aggression. His contributions were, however, always relevant to the content of the session, and could usually be constructively used by the facilitators to emphasise relevant learning or to provoke further discussion amongst the class. Even Dylan, who had a history of addiction and problems concentrating, reported enjoying the programme and actively contributed on a regular basis. It had taken a few weeks for him to feel comfortable:

> I did not really say much at first, man, just liked to know what other people were saying and all that, and then I started speaking a couple of weeks later. But aye, it [the programme] was worth it, definitely.

Engagement was high, and did not vary greatly from week to week or topic to topic, or even from man to man in terms of level, if not style, of engagement. Towards the end of the 10-week programme, there were several discussions initiated by the men around why they were not able to begin the programme again once they finished that programme. Most of them expressed a desire to "keep on coming along". Indeed, the facilitators set up a "keeping in touch" group for which take-up has been high according to post-fieldwork reports from the facilitators to the author.

Factors facilitating successful implementation

Relationship between facilitators and participants

The positive relationships between the facilitators and the participants was regarded by Barnardo's Scotland as a key potential mechanism for change. As a Barnardo's manager said:

> If we can do that for those dads, then they can do that for their children 'cause they know that it feels good to have somebody be positive. If we can help someone to know how it feels to have somebody else thinking about you, then can they open up something for their little one.

It was regarded as essential that the programme was delivered in a conducive context where the facilitators demonstrated respect for the participants of the course and built up nurturing relationships.

The two Parenting Officers recruited to deliver the programme were very different in their demographic profile and in their manner and style. They were both Prison Officers with many years' experience of working with the men in the halls; one had worked for the SPS since leaving university and the other had come to the SPS after being in the armed forces. One was male, the other female; one had children and a spouse, the other had a partner but no children. One was very open and willing to discuss personal issues with the young men, the other was much more private though did share some specific examples relating to parenthood. Both used humour in delivering the programme and were adept at managing the young men's behaviour, keeping them focused on the task at hand, whilst being respectful to them. While it was clear who was in charge and clear boundaries were maintained, the Parenting Officers interacted with them on first name terms and chatted with them about many aspects of their lives, treating them as much more than simply "prisoners".

One Parenting Officer expressed frustration on one or more occasions around the "heavy handedness" of other Prison Officers in their treatment of the young men around their participation in the parenting intervention. For example, it was observed that during a family visit one of the men was taken away from his partner and children as it was suspected his partner had handed him drugs. The Parenting Officer felt that there was no need to have "marched him off" to be searched when his child was present, and that the situation—whilst it had to be addressed—could have been dealt with in a subtle way. While the two Parenting Officers were very clearly inculcated into the culture of the YOI, having worked as Prison Officers for many years, they explicitly recognised (and it was implicit in their observed behaviour) that a slightly different relationship was required in their role as Parenting Officers, and were protective of the programme participants when they felt that "normal prison culture" was impinging on the more caring ethos surrounding the parenting programme.

The ways in which the facilitators endeavoured to build this different sort of relationship with the participants, winning their trust, included calling them by their first names, and introducing themselves by their first names; offering them cups of coffee and snacks; giving them positive personal feedback; having quite lengthy conversations with them about parts of their lives which had nothing to do with their status as prisoners; and sharing some aspects of their own lives with the men. Much of this had been encouraged by Barnardo's when the partnership was first initiated. As one of the Barnardo's staff said:

> it's that relation of currency, and I think perhaps in the hall mentalities you [the Prison Officer] don't tell them [the men] anything, but I think you have to. If you're going to be part of somebody's life and meeting their child and their partner, and they're letting you in, you need to give something.

From what was observed, for this study several months after the working partnership between the SPS and Barnardo's had begun, the Parenting Officers had great respect for the men, even when individual men were exhibiting challenging behaviour as happened from time to time.

For the Barnardo's facilitator, it was perhaps more "natural" to develop such a respectful relationship with the young men than it was for these Parenting Officers who had worked in the halls of prisons for many years. Although this was the first time she had delivered a programme within a prison, and she had undertaken much more work with mothers than with fathers, she was very experienced in delivering parenting work to vulnerable populations, and well versed in what she called "reaching out to the most disadvantaged families", a central tenet of Barnardo's work.

The men did notice, and appreciate, efforts to build relationships in these ways. As Dino said:

> see in the halls they're [Prison Officers] not like that, but up here, aye. Tom and Heather are sound man, they're all right.

Harry said:

> Everyone that was part of the course was good people ... if they weren't I wouldn't have paid any attention, I wouldn't have cared, I wouldn't have bothered with it. Respect goes a long way.

Relationships between the men

In their conscious quest to create respectful caring relationships with the men, it was hoped that a by-product would be the men developing caring relationships with each other as the parenting classroom became a place where all within it would listen to each other, respect would prevail, and it would be free of aggression and conflict and safe for all to express their feelings and thoughts.

The opening session included the men setting ground rules. They were encouraged to come up with some rules that would create a safe and caring atmosphere within the classroom: what is said in the room is confidential; no judging each other; no *personal* banter; and respect each other.

When the Parenting Officers were aware that there had been conflict between individual men in the past they worked to try to ensure that this was left behind within the parenting classroom. For example, Saul and Jimmy had a history of conflict in their community, before imprisonment, but were in the same parenting group. The Parenting Officers did some conciliation work with them before the course began.

When racist, homophobic, sexist or similar remarks were made within the classroom, they were usually challenged, in a firm but respectful way, by the facilitators. Jimmy, for example, often made derogative remarks about his partner, the mother of his children. Over the weeks, it was observed that these were challenged not only by the facilitators, but by the other men. When Dylan made homophobic remarks, with violent connotations, his statements were deemed unacceptable and were unpacked by the facilitators. They talked him through how such comments may make others feel. Barnardo's staff had, initially, had concerns that challenging the men in this way may not be something the Parenting Officers were easily able to do. A manager reported that Barnardo's Equality and Diversity training had been undertaken by the Parenting Officers, in addition to SPS training, and from what was observed the Parenting Officers appeared to be comfortable with such challenging.

For both the groups observed, there was little or no conflict between the men, though the amount of "banter"—which could be challenging for the facilitators to manage—varied depending on which particular individuals were there for each session. Generally, it was observed that the bigger the group, the more high spirited it was, but even at the times of peak liveliness, the young men managed to stay on task and to put their interactions with each other aside to focus on the session itself. However, since this fieldwork was undertaken, the facilitators have reported that there have been a small number of groups which have failed to work well together, and where engagement has been compromised as a result.

The classroom climate

The classroom climate is a product of the relationships discussed above, as well as being shaped by things such as the aesthetic environment, discussed below. Buston (2018) discusses in detail how a caring, sharing climate was created in the deliveries observed, a climate which allowed the men to show their softer side in the parenting classroom. Being a father and showing emotion in relation to one's children and partner was an acceptable masculine identity within the classroom.

As well as the work done by the facilitators to foster conducive relationships between themselves and the men, and between the men, there were also other nurturing efforts made. The Barnardo's facilitator brought in milk each day, and fruit or biscuits, and the classroom was stocked with coffee, tea and juice. If the men talked about missing particular items of food, she would sometimes buy these. As Dino said:

> we do appreciate that [provision of food and drink] because we don't get decent, a lot of folk don't get a lot of money sent in so they don't go and buy a bag of Nescafe 'cause it's 4.50, a lot of the boys are like that "no, I can't pay that for a bag", so they appreciate it. And biscuits, you don't get biscuits like that in here. Feel looked after, aye.

The room itself was light and bright, there were beanbags to sit on as well as the more traditional tables and chairs, and at times the radio was switched on to provide background music. One of the Barnardo's managers described it:

> they've got this amazing new room. It's beautiful, this whole activities building is just a different world. It's brightly coloured, just bright colours everywhere, like nice images. It's so lovely and apparently the dads all said, 'cause they were in it last week I think, and they were like "oh, it's like a college. It's like being in a college". Which is what you want. You want them to have a different sense [there than in the rest of the prison], a sense of learning.

Content and methods

What was delivered, and *how* it was delivered, also facilitated ongoing engagement. Observations suggested the men were open to learning about a variety of topics, and liked to discuss, participate in quizzes, and undertake practical exercises such as cooking and making cards. This was corroborated by the interview data with the young men. The facilitators appeared to be very good at gauging if boredom was rising, and engagement was waning, and were flexible in their delivery of particular segments, knowing when to cease or change pace or direction. It was observed that when concentration flagged, board games were brought out or there was informal discussion over coffee. The Parenting Officer and Barnardo's facilitator were, overall, much more successful in engaging the men than outside facilitators, though this varied. The men were fascinated by a visitor from the Fire Brigade, for example, who talked about fire safety in a humorous, animated way, but were bored—the observations and interview data suggest—by a member of the prison health staff who came in to talk about passive smoking and the dangers of drugs. The manner of the visitor, and the extent to which s/he appeared to be able to relate to the young men, had a bigger impact than the content itself.

The men reported enjoying arts and crafts activities, this was evident from observations also. They usually had an ongoing craft project, for example making a Mother's Day card or a book for their child. Often at the end of a morning or afternoon, when they were tired of doing other things, these were brought out. During the sessions which were observed, some of the men asked that they take the items back to their cells to work on. A mix of activities during each session worked best: a discussion session followed by a game; or skills-based work followed by some arts and crafts.

The prison context

Both the financial and opportunity cost of, and the effort involved in, attending an intervention such as this must be considered. If this was offered in the community, the young fathers might miss valuable leisure time if they were to attend. It might cost them money to get to the venue by bus or taxi, and require effort to plan and get themselves there at the same time each week. In the prison, however, there is little to do during the day. Most of those on the programme reported that they would have been in their cell, trying to fill their time, if they were not at the parenting session. The men needed to make very little effort to attend the classes; all that was required was that they wait for the 'prison route' (when prisoners are escorted by Prison Officers from one part of the prison to another) to take them from their hall to the parenting classroom. From the point of view of those implementing the course, therefore, the men were very accessible. The facilitators reported that the men could be approached at induction or in their cells where they could be asked to identify themselves as fathers, and that they also had access to other sources of information about the men's fatherhood status. These young men, imprisoned in the Scottish context, were drug and alcohol free when incarcerated; many would not be in the community.

In terms of the men's motivation, some of them mentioned that, when they had first been approached about the programme at least, they had thought their attendance might "count for something" with social work, or in terms of an early release. None, however, seemed to then continue to attend simply so it looked good in this way. Timmy, for example, who had not yet secured access to his baby and reported desperately wanting this contact, explained that his prime motivation for attending the course was to show social work that he really did want to be a father to his child; he felt this commitment "proved" this in a way he was not able to do with his words alone. His reports, and what was observed, suggested that he wanted to learn during the programme so that when/if he did get access he would know how to look after and interact with his child:

> see as long as it's going to get social work off my back, to make them see that I'm not just putting a front on 'cause I'm in the jail doing this. I'm doing it just to show them that I am trying, I *do* want to be a dad.

Some of the men also talked about a general desire to make themselves better people during their prison sentence, which may also have been the prime motivation for first attending for some. Overall, though, there was a sense amongst the men that this programme might actually help them to be better fathers, something that they all said they wanted. Many of them had had traumatic upbringings; this often became increasingly apparent as the programme progressed, and they wanted to know how to provide the loving and caring environment for their child(ren) that they had not had.

Barriers to successful implementation

There were barriers and challenges which compromised, or threatened to compromise, individual men's ongoing engagement from time to time. Barnardo's had had to undertake considerable amounts of "behind the scenes" work as a foundation for the intervention delivery in the prison. Introducing "new ways" of working to the YOI was challenging. Sometimes these new ways of working, seen by Barnardo's as a necessary foundation for implementation of the intervention, were threatened. For example, one of the Barnardo's staff members described the resistance of prison staff when the facilitator bought one of the participants a birthday card and cake on his 21st birthday. She felt that while the Barnardo's staff member saw it as an "obvious" aspect of nurturing, core to the intervention, prison staff saw it as "alien". As one of Barnardo's managers said:

It's a very difficult environment to do this in. Not because people are deliberately obstructive, people just don't work in that way ... I don't think it's a malicious thing ... . It's just that they don't know [this way of working]. Stuff that we [Barnardo's] just do without thinking and I think "oh, they'll just know how to do that", and they don't.

The Barnardo's staff were very reflective about their ways of working, and how the ethos of Barnardo's as an organisation was very different to that of SPS. Interviews and conversations with these staff described the groundwork undertaken at the early stages of intervention delivery. During the fieldwork, however, there were several instances where organisational value clashes became apparent. These usually stemmed from differences relating to how the young men were viewed, with the ethos of Barnardo's dictating they should be treated as equals, and valued in an unconditional way, but the institutional mores of the prison service not always facilitating this to the extent Barnardo's would find acceptable in order to maintain the trust necessary to fully engage the men on an ongoing basis in the intervention work.

There were also social work and other issues around the men's status as fathers which were outside the control of those delivering the programme, but that sometimes compromised the men's willingness to engage. The men sometimes felt frustrated with the facilitators if social work meetings around access were slow to organise, or decisions did not go their way, and were then less amenable to participating in classroom sessions. During one of the observed family visits Timmy was expecting his ex-girlfriend and baby but they did not arrive. A Prison Officer had not been available to escort Timmy back to the halls once it was apparent that his child was not coming, so he had had to sit with the other men and their families as they interacted. He was visibly upset during this time. The Parenting Officers reported how they had to undertake one-to-one counselling with Timmy following this to ensure that he felt able to complete the rest of the course following this incident. Interviews and conversations suggested that he, the facilitators, and the other men who had received visits that day felt very uncomfortable with him having to sit through the visits from other partners and children.

There were groups, not observed during the fieldwork but talked about by the facilitators, where members failed to work well together, making delivery and the facilitation of engagement difficult. This was usually, it was reported, down to the presence of one disruptive individual. Many of the young men in the YOI had problems concentrating and/or reading and writing, but the responses to the programme by those with the most extreme difficulties in these areas have sometimes made it difficult for their class-mates to engage. Barnardo's are very clear that these men, amongst the most vulnerable in the prison, should not be excluded from the group, but it is recognised that these individuals can compromise others' engagement. Staff report working on solutions to ensure that these men can be included, and feel able to engage, and do not hijack the experiences of others.

Discussion and conclusions

The paper has focused on the recruitment, retention and engagement of young incarcerated men in a prison-based parenting intervention for fathers, elucidating processes of implementation and identifying facilitating factors and barriers. Qualitative data collection has utilised a range of methods to collect data from, and with, a number of incarcerated men and staff involved in managing and delivering the intervention, over a prolonged period of time, and spanning different deliveries of the same programme delivered by different facilitators. Framework analysis was undertaken on the integrated data set. Whilst adding specifically to the very sparse literature on engaging incarcerated young fathers in parenting work, the findings have transferability to other under-researched areas. They will be particularly useful for those working in the prison setting implementing any social intervention with inmates, and also have utility for those working in the community implementing parenting and family work with marginalised young fathers.

This intervention is an example of a parenting intervention which successfully recruited, retained and engaged fathers. Furthermore, it successfully recruited, retained and engaged marginalised, vulnerable, traditionally "hard-to-reach" fathers. Why was it successful?

First, trust and respect were key in motivating engagement, concurring with existing literature (Axford et al., 2012; Katz et al., 2007; Pfitzner, Humphreys, & Hegarty, 2017). Those delivering the programme invested time and effort in building relationships with parents. Particularly in the prison environment, where there is a general mistrust towards prison service staff, the Parenting Officers, in their prison uniforms and as SPS representatives, were successful in winning the young men's trust through their manner. The involvement of an outside facilitator, in civilian clothes and clearly not employed by the prison service, probably helped. Her skills in delivering parenting work and forming such trusting relationships over a number of years were key.

Second, the practical aspects involved facilitated engagement (Pfitzner et al., 2017). A programme delivered, almost literally, on the doorstep of the men's cells with no financial cost and little opportunity cost involved in attendance will attract and retain the men more than one where costs are high in these terms.

Third, that this programme focused specifically on fathers, in the context of an all male prison, seems important, though this is hard to draw conclusions around as there is no comparison of a mixed sex prison parenting programme. Certainly these men seemed to find commonalities with each other. It was implicit in much of their interaction that they came from similar communities, had similar backgrounds, and were of similar socio-economic status. They were all at the same life stage and their children were all very young. Furthermore, there was an understanding amongst them that they had taken a similar path in life, ending, for now, there in the jail, and they appeared to have similar knowledge, attitudes and behaviours with regard to parenting as well as other topics. As young fathers, they sometimes talked about how they perceived they were being judged as deficient in some ways by others, appearing to share an identity as fathers who cared but who had to overcome some barriers in order to be seen as "proper parents". They generally saw their role as fathers as being distinct from that of mothers. The homogeneity of the group in all of these respects meant it was fairly straightforward for the facilitators to ensure that content was relevant and of interest to all members of the group, a characteristic of effective social interventions (Bronte-Tinkew et al., 2008). Indeed, this homogeneity facilitated high levels of engagement both because group members were able to bond together and because approaches and content could be targeted to the needs and interests of all the men. Available evidence does indicate that the involvement of both parents in interventions is the optimal way forward (Lundahl et al., 2008; Ramchandani & Iles, 2014) but opportunities such as this where groups of otherwise hard-to-reach men can be successfully involved in and engaged with targeted parenting work should be grasped.

Fourth, the men's desires to be "good fathers" should be noted. Young incarcerated men appear to aspire to being caring fathers: warm, sensitive, attentive, protective of their child, and spending time with and supporting him/her (Buston, 2010; Buston, O'Brien, & Maxwell, in preparation). All of the fathers participating in the two deliveries observed for this study said that they wanted to be good fathers. Nearly all of them reported unhappy childhoods and wanted to be there for their child(ren) in the way their biological father had not been (Buston et al., in preparation). Furthermore, most recognised that the way they had been fathered was a potential barrier to them fathering in positive ways. They wanted to be good fathers, and they recognised that attending this parenting course could be helpful in facilitating this.

This study was a process evaluation. It did not focus on outcomes, instead seeking to examine how the intervention was implemented. It was very much formative, and exploratory, work, designed to be able to feedback to Barnardo's on the initial deliveries of the programme with this population, suggesting mechanisms which might lead to it being effective across the men, while identifying barriers and facilitating factors to it being delivered, and received, as intended. The next step would be to conduct a rigorous outcome evaluation. The results reported in this paper, and those to be reported elsewhere (Buston, in press; Buston et al., in preparation) will form a solid foundation for this work.

Recent work has noted that engaging with fathers is one of the least well-explored and articulated aspects of parenting interventions (La Placa & Corlyon, 2014; Panter-Brick et al., 2014), and, indeed, of family services generally (Scourfield et al., 2014). This paper contributes to better understanding some of the mechanisms which facilitate engagement. Findings highlight the need to look beyond content in understanding why any parenting programme, in the prison or in the community, might successfully engage its participants in a sustained way. These fathers very much appreciated the classroom context in which the programme was delivered; a caring, sharing, nurturing ethos within the parenting classroom will facilitate engagement amongst similar groups of marginalised young fathers within the community also, and there are lessons to be learned for engaging fathers in family services more generally. The work supports assertions that particular parents are not, by dint of who they are, necessarily "hard-to-reach" but instead it may be that particular interventions and services are hard [for them] to access (Davies, 2016). The prison is an opportunity for delivering parenting programmes to incarcerated fathers, an opportunity that should be grasped as it can be a highly conducive setting for such work, albeit with institutional challenges, some of which threatened to compromise aspects of engagement for this programme (Miller et al., 2014).

Acknowledgements

Thanks to Barnardo's Scotland and the Scottish Prison Service who facilitated collaborative working on this study. Thank you also to the young men who welcomed me into the parenting classroom, as well as the staff from Barnardo's and SPS who will not be named to preserve their anonymity.

Disclosure statement

No potential conflict of interest was reported by the author.

Funding

The study was funded by the Medical Research Council [MC_UU_12017/11 and SPHSU11]. The core fieldwork took place between January and May 2015.

References

Axford, N., Lehtonen, M., Kaoukji, D., Tobin, K., & Berry, V. (2012). Engaging parents in parenting programs: Lessons from research and practice. *Children and Youth Services Review, 34*, 2061–2071.

Barlow, J., Smailagic, N., Bennett, C., Huband, N., Jones, H., & Coren, E. (2011). Individual and group based parenting programmes for improving psychosocial outcomes for teenage parents and their children. *Cochrane Database of Systematic Reviews* (3). Art. No.: CD002964. doi: 10.1002/14651858.CD002964.pub2

Bayley, J., Wallace, L. M., & Choudhry, K. (2009). Fathers and parenting programmes: Barriers and best practice. *Community Practitioner, 82*, 28–31.

Berlyn, C., Wise, S., & Soriano, G. (2008). *Engaging fathers in child and family services. Participation, perceptions and good practice*. Canberra: University of New South Wales, National Evaluation Consortium, Social Policy Research Centre.

Bronte-Tinkew, J., Carrano, J., Allen, T., Bowie, L., Mbawa, K., & Matthews, G. (2008). Elements of promising practice for fatherhood programs: Evidence-based research findings on programs for fathers. Gaithersburg, MD 20877: National Responsible Fatherhood Clearinghouse for U.S. Department of Health and Human Services Office of Family Assistance.

Buston, K. (2010). Experiences of, and attitudes towards, pregnancy and fatherhood amongst incarcerated young male offenders: Findings from a qualitative study. *Social Science and Medicine, 71*, 2212–2218.

Buston, K. (2018). Inside the prison parenting classroom: Caring, sharing and the softer side of masculinity. In M. Maycock, & K. Hunt (Eds.), *New perspectives on prison masculnities* (pp. 277–306). London: Palgrave.

Buston, K., O'Brien, R., & Maxwell, K. (in preparation). They much you up, your mum and dad: Arguing the case for more, targetted, parenting intervention work with reference to inter-generational transmission of parenting.

Buston, K., Parkes, A., Thomson, H., Wight, D., & Fenton, C. (2012). Parenting interventions for male young offenders: A review of evidence on what works. *Journal of Adolescence, 35*, 731–742.

Cowan, P. A., Cowan, C. P., Pruett, M. K., Pruett, K., & Wong, J. J. (2009). Promoting fathers' engagement with children: Preventive interventions for low-income families. *Journal of Marriage and Family, 71*, 663–679.

Davies, L. (2016). Are young fathers "hard to reach"? understanding the importance of relationship building and service sustainability. *Journal of Children's Services, 11*, 317–329.

Ferguson, H. (2016). Patterns of engagement and non-engagement of young fathers in early intervention and safeguarding work. *Social Policy and Society, 15*, 99–111.

Fletcher, R., & Visser, A. (2008). Faciliating father engagement: The role of family relationship centres. *Journal of Family Studies, 14*, 53–64.

Flouri, E., & Buchanan, A. (2002). Father involvement in childhood and trouble with the police in adolescence: Findings from the 1958 British cohort. *Journal of Interpersonal Violence, 17*, 689–701.

Flouri, E., & Buchanan, A. (2003). The role of father involvement in children's later mental health. *Journal of Adolescence, 26*, 63–78.

Flouri, E., & Buchanan, A. (2004). Early father's and mother's involvement and child's later educational outcomes. *British Journal of Educational Psychology, 74*, 141–153.

Flouri, E., Buchanan, A., & Bream, V. (2002). Adolescents' perceptions of their fathers' involvement: Significance to school attitudes. *Psychology in the Schools, 39*, 575–582.

Gale, N. K., Heath, G., Cameron, E., Rashid, S., & Redwood, S. (2013). Using the framework method for the analysis of qualitative data in multi-disciplinary health research. *BMC Medical Research Methodology, 13*, 117. doi:10.1186/1471-2288-13-117

Katz, I., Corlyon, J., La Placa, V., & Hunter, S. (2007). *The relationship between parenting and poverty*. York: Joseph Rowntree Foundation.

Katz, I., La Placa, V., & Hunter, S. (2007). *Barrers to inclusion and successful engagement of parents in mainstream services*. York: Joseph Rowntree Foundation.

Kazura, K. (2001). Family programming for incarcerated parents: A needs assessment among inmates. *Journal of Offender Rehabilitation, 32*, 67–83.

Kim, M., Kang, S., Yee, B., Shim, S., & Chung, M. (2016). Paternal involvement and early infant neurodevelopment: The mediation role of maternal parenting stress. *BMC Pediatrics, 16*, 212. doi:10.1186/s12887-016-0747-y.

Kroll, M., Carson, C., Redshaw, M., & Quigley, M. A. (2016). Early father involvement and subsequent child behaviour at ages 3, 5 and 7 years: Prospective analysis of the UK millenium cohort study. *Plos One, 11*(9), e0162339. http://doi.org/10 1371/journal.pone.0162339.

La Placa, V., & Corlyon, J. (2014). Barriers to inclusion and successful engagement of parents in mainstream services: Evidence and research. *Journal of Children's Services, 9*, 220–234.

Lindsay, G., Davies, H., Band, S., Cullen, M. A., Cullen, S., & Strand, S. (2008). Parenting early intervention pathfinder: Research report RW054. London: DCSF.

Lundahl, B. W., Tollefson, D., Risser, H., & Lovejoy, M. C. (2008). A meta-analysis of father involvement in parent training. *Research on Social Work Practice, 18*, 97–106.

Macmillan, C. (2005). Public health initiative at a young offenders institute. *Community Practitioner, 78*, 397–399.

Magill-Evans, J., Harrison, M. J., Rempel, G., & Slater, L. (2006). Interventions with fathers of young children: Systematic literature review. *Journal of Advanced Nursing, 55*, 248–264.

Maxwell, N., Scourfield, J., Featherstone, B., Holland, S., & Tolman, R. (2012). Engaging fathers in child welfare services: A narrative review of recent research evidence. *Child & Family Social Work, 17*, 160–169.

Miller, A. L., Weston, L. E., Perryman, J., Horwitz, T., Franzen, S., & Cochran, S. (2014). Parenting while incarcerated: Tailoring the strengthening families program for use with jailed mothers. *Children and Youth Services Review, 44*, 163–170.

Moran, P., Ghate, D., & van der Merwe, A. (2004). *What works in parenting support? A review of the international evidence*. London: Policy Research Bureau.

Nurse, A. (2001). The structure of the juvenile prison - constructing the inmate father. *Youth & Society, 32*, 360–394.

O'Brien, R., Hunt, K., & Hart, G. (2005). "It's caveman stuff but that is to a certain extent how guys still operate": men's accounts of masculinity and hep seeking. *Social Science & Medicine, 61*, 503–516.

Panter-Brick, C., Burgess, A., Eggerman, M., McAllister, F., Pruett, K., & Leckman, J. F. (2014). Practitioner review: Engaging fathers - recommendations for a game change in parenting interventions based on a systematic review of the global evidence. *Journal of Child Psychology and Psychiatry, 55*, 1187–1212.

Pfitzner, N., Humphreys, C., & Hegarty, K. (2017). Research review: Engaging men: A multi-level model to support father engagement. *Child & Family Social Work, 22*, 537–547.

Philip, G., & O'Brien, M. (2012). *Supporting fathers after separation or divorce: Evidence and insights*. Norwich: University of East Anglia Centre for Research on the Child and Family.

Ramchandani, P., & Iles, J. (2014). Commentary: Getting fathers into parenting programmes - a reflection on panter-brock et al. (2014). *The Journal of Child Psychology and Psychiatry*, *55*, 1213–1214.

Ritchie, J., & Lewis, J. (2003). *Qualitative research practice: A guide for social science students and researchers*. London: Sage.

Roberts, A., Onwumere, J., Forrester, A., Huddy, V., Byrne, M., Campbell, C. ... Valmaggia, L. (2016). Family intervention in a prison enviroment: A systematic literature review. *Criminal Behaviour and Mental Health*, 326–340. doi:10.1002/cbm.2001

Ross, N., Church, S., Hill, M., Seaman, P., & Roberts, T. (2012). The perspectives of young men and their teenage partners on maternity and health services during pregnancy and early parenthood. *Children and Society*, *26*, 304–315.

Saldana, J. (2013). *The coding manual for qualitative researchers*. London: Sage.

Scottish Prison Service. (2013). *Unlocking potential: Report of the scottish prison service organisational review*. Edinburgh: Scottish Prison Service.

Scourfield, J., Yi Cheung, S., & Macdonald, G. (2014). Working with fathers to improve children's well-being: Results of a survey exploring service provision and intervention approach in the UK. *Children and Youth Services Review*, *43*, 40–50.

Smith, T. K., Duggan, A., Bair-Merritt, M. H., & Cox, G. (2012). Systematic review of fathers' involvement in programmes for the primary prevention of child maltreatment. *Child Abuse Review*, *21*, 237–254.

Allowing Imprisoned Fathers to Parent: Maximising the Potential Benefits of Prison based Parenting Programmes

David Hayes ⓘ, Michelle Butler ⓘ, John Devaney ⓘ and Andrew Percy ⓘ

ABSTRACT

During imprisonment, fathers are separated from their families and contact is limited. When delivering a prison based parenting programme, providing an opportunity to rehearse newly acquired parenting skills can be key for mastering the performance of these skills and using these skills to improve father-child relationships. This paper takes an in-depth look at how one parenting programme in Northern Ireland sought to overcome this challenge by providing additional opportunities to parent via increased telephone contact and special family friendly visits. Using a combination of in-depth interviews and observations, how fathers and their families responded to this increased contact is explored, as well as the extent to which this increased contact facilitated the acquisition of the parenting skills being taught on the programme. It is argued that while prison based parenting programmes can improve parenting skills and father-child relationships, their potential long-term effectiveness may be limited by wider prison policies, procedures and practices surrounding prison visitation, telephone access and the progression of fathers following the completion of such programmes. Recommendations and suggestions for future practice are offered.

Nowadays, imprisonment is generally used to punish wrongdoing by depriving an individual of their liberty and separating them from loved ones (Garland, 1990). However, the potential for this separation to negatively affect the development and wellbeing of children has become increasingly documented in countries such as the U.S.A., U.K., Australia, New Zealand and Denmark (Flynn & Eriksson, 2015; Foster & Hagan, 2009; Hagan & Foster, 2012; Wildeman, 2009). While the majority of research on parental imprisonment has focused on mothers, there is a growing recognition of the need to look at the impact of fathers' imprisonment, as the majority of those imprisoned internationally are men (Walmsley, 2016). For those with positive father–child relationships, this separation can weaken and disrupt father–child interactions and increase adverse outcomes for children (Dennison, Smallbone, & Occhipinti, 2017; Sharratt, 2014). Examples of such adverse outcomes that have been identified in research conducted in the U.S.A. and the U.K. include reduced well-being, poorer educational attainment, criminality, social exclusion, mental health problems and behavioural difficulties (Foster & Hagan, 2009; Hagan & Dinovitzer, 1999; Murray & Murray, 2010; Wakefield & Wildeman, 2011; Wildeman, 2014). Prison based parenting programmes in the U.S.A., the U.K. and Australia have sought to mitigate the negative effects of separation by increasing family contact and improving parenting skills (Hoffmann, Byrd, & Kightlinger, 2010; Meek, 2007; Newman, Fowler, & Cashin, 2011). However, one of the challenges faced by such programmes is how prison policies, procedures and practices (for example, the lack of access to toys or games during standard prison visits) can curtail opportunities to rehearse parenting skills, as well as the amount and quality of contact fathers have with their children (Dennison et al., 2017; Hutton, 2016; Sharratt, 2014).

This paper takes an in-depth look at how one prison based parenting programme in Northern Ireland sought to overcome these difficulties by providing additional opportunities for contact between imprisoned fathers and their children. Responses to this increased contact are examined to explore if it helped improve father–child relationships and the acquisition of parenting skills. It is argued that while prison based parenting programmes can enhance parenting skills and contribute to improvements in father–child relationships, this is dependent on the extent fathers are allowed to use these skills while imprisoned to improve relationships with their children.

Prison based parenting programmes

There are a range of parenting programmes offered in prison (Buston, Parkes, Thomson, Wight, & Fenton, 2012; Hoffmann et al., 2010; Loper & Tuerk, 2006; Newman et al., 2011). These programmes vary in their format but usually incorporate parenting classes, child friendly visiting arrangements, increased family contact and support for family members (Barnardo's, 2015; Barr et al., 2011; Barr et al., 2014; Boswell, Poland, & Price, 2010; Buston et al., 2012; Meek, 2007; Purvis, 2013). Research in the U.S.A., U.K. and Australia indicates that these programmes are largely beneficial, at least in the short term, resulting in increased parenting skills, confidence and ability to understand children's needs, as well as improved family communication and relationships (Boswell et al., 2010; Buston et al., 2012; Loper & Tuerk, 2006; McCrudden, Braiden, McCormack, Sloan, & Treacy, 2014; Purvis, 2013). Nevertheless, the fundamental challenge for these programmes is the separation of imprisoned fathers from their children and how fathers can maintain contact with their children while imprisoned (Buston et al., 2012; Loper & Tuerk, 2006; Purvis, 2013).

Both U.S. and European research indicates that telephone calls, letters and visits are the most common ways in which imprisoned parents maintain contact with their children (La Vigne, Naser, Brooks, & Castro, 2005; Sharratt, 2014), yet prisons in different jurisdictions and at different security levels vary in the policies, practices and procedures they use to govern visitation, telephone access and letter-writing (Hutton, 2016; La Vigne et al., 2005; Sharratt, 2014). These differences partially explain why the effect of parental imprisonment on child adverse outcomes can vary between jurisdictions, with some jurisdictions experiencing worse outcomes (e.g. the U.K.) than others (e.g. the Netherlands or Sweden) (Besemer, van der Geest, Murray, Bijleveld, & Farrington, 2011; Hutton, 2016; Murray, Janson, & Farrington, 2007). For example, crowded prison visiting areas and restrictions on movement and physical contact can create an artificial environment for father–child interactions, resulting in strained communications and poor quality inter-actions (Dennison et al., 2017; Hutton, 2016; Sharratt, 2014). Over time, this type of contact can weaken social bonds and contribute to relationship breakdown (Dennison et al., 2017). For this reason, prisons which adopt child friendly visiting arrangements are believed to be more effective at protecting children's wellbeing and building positive father–child relationships (Dennison et al., 2017; Poehlmann, Dallaire, Loper, & Shear, 2010). Moreover, maintaining contact is not only important for children but it also pro-vides fathers with an opportunity to rehearse their parenting skills and reaffirm their iden-tity as a parent (Dennison et al., 2017).

Skill acquisition is considered an important component of many skills based pro-grammes and is generally understood as a three-stage process involving: 1) acquiring new knowledge; 2) consolidating knowledge through practice; and 3) automating the per-formance of new skills through frequent use and rehearsal (Proctor & Dutta, 1995). Infre-quent use of new skills can lead to a failure to accurately perform and retain these skills, increasing the likelihood of new skills being lost and forgotten (Kim, Ritter, & Koubek, 2013; Proctor & Dutta, 1995). Within parenting programmes, encouraging parents to practice newly acquired skills has been found to improve skill retention, performance and child outcomes (Bronte-Tinkew et al., 2008; Stokes et al., 2016). Given the separation imprisoned parents experience from their children, opportunities to practise newly acquired parenting skills may be essential if these skills are to be successfully retained and mastered. In this study, how one Northern Ireland prison based parenting programme at Maghaberry Prison, the Families Matter programme, sought to overcome these difficul-ties is explored.

The present paper

The political conflict in Northern Ireland has played a considerable role in shaping the Northern Ireland prison system with the challenges posed by political prisoners, protests, hunger strikes and violence, historically contributing to a more restrictive, security focused regime, especially within Maghaberry Prison (Butler, 2016). While recent reforms have sought to transform the prison service, Maghaberry Prison remains the highest security category prison in Northern Ireland and political prisoners continue to be held there (Butler, 2016). The findings presented in this paper are drawn from a project investigating the design, rationale and implementation of the Families Matter programme, as well as how fathers, families and staff responded to the programme (see Butler, Hayes, Devaney, & Percy, 2015). This project examined the strengths and weaknesses of the pro-gramme design, its implementation and its ability to reduce some of the negative effects associated with parental imprisonment (see Butler et al., 2015). This paper draws on these findings to provide an in-depth exploration of the level of family contact participants experienced prior to and during the programme and how this contact affected family relationships and parenting skill acquisition. At the time of the research, the Families Matter programme was an adult male -17-week residential parenting programme based at Maghaberry Prison, Northern Ireland. The programme was jointly developed by Bar-nardo's Northern Ireland and the Northern Ireland Prison Service and opened to fathers on remand and sentenced to long and short periods of custody (see Butler et al.,

2015 for further information about the programme). Assessments were also conducted with fathers to assess their parenting skills and quality of parental relationships before joining the programme. The programme sought to improve father–child relationships by increasing the frequency and quality of father–child contact and strengthen parenting skills via participation in parenting classes and a range of other educational and family focused activities. The frequency and quality of family contact was increased by providing fathers with extra telephone access and special monthly family-friendly visits, in addition to the normal prison visits that were available. Fathers and their families were only allowed to avail themselves of these additional opportunities for contact during the programme and returned to pre-programme levels of contact upon programme completion. This paper focuses specifically on how the additional opportunities for contact were responded to by fathers and their families to explore if it helped improve relationships and the acquisition of parenting skills.

Methods

Research design

A mixed methods approach combining observations and interviews was used to examine the design, rationale, implementation and effect of programme participation. Ten days of non-participant observation was conducted to observe programme content and delivery, as well as how fathers and their families responded to the programme. Observations were deemed an essential component of the methodology as the 'what works' literature indicates that how programmes are designed and delivered can influence their effectiveness (Andrews & Dowden, 2005; Hollin, 1995; Lipsey, 1995). In-depth semi-structured interviews were conducted with 42 individuals, consisting of 18 fathers, 7 family members and 17 staff (please contact the authors for a copy of the interview schedules used). All bar one of the fathers agreed to participate in the study. Fathers were interviewed twice (half way through the programme and on completion) to investigate if responses changed over time. Observations were also ongoing during this time, allowing interview responses to be compared with observed behaviour. Family members and staff were interviewed once on programme completion.

Procedure

Ethics approval was obtained from three ethics committees; Queen's University Belfast, the Northern Ireland Prison Service and Barnardo's UK. Full security clearance was obtained for the research team, and relevant professional guidelines and protocols were followed.

Potential participants were identified and recruited through their involvement in the Families Matter programme and were informed of the study using a combination of verbal announcements, information sessions, posters and information sheets. The voluntary nature of the research was stressed and potential participants were advised that they could refuse to answer questions or withdraw from the study at any stage, without any negative consequences. In addition, the limits to confidentiality and anonymity were outlined and all were aware that disclosures of abuse, staff malpractice, harm to self/others and attempts to escape would be reported to a relevant authority. Due to the small number of people participating in the programme, potentially identifying information has been removed in an attempt to protect participants' confidentiality and anonymity.

Data analysis

A theory of action approach was used to analyse and interpret the observations. This involves attempting to make links between events occurring on the programme and their actual and potential effect on individuals (Friedman & Antal, 2005; Parson, Shils, & Smelser, 2001). The interview data were analysed using NVivo and interpreted using thematic analysis. Thematic analysis is a qualitative methodology used to identify, analyse and report patterns or themes in qualitative data (Braun & Clarke, 2006). This method of analysis was used to identify recurring themes in the participants' perceptions and experiences of family contact, as well as how family contact may affect family relationships and the acquisition of parenting skills. Quotes from the interviews with fathers, family members and staff have been chosen for inclusion in the findings section as they exemplify the themes being discussed. Data triangulation was used to crosscheck the findings emerging from the interviews with those from the observations, to ensure that the claims, conclusions and recommendations drawn from the research were accurate and supported by the data (Bryman, 2008).

Findings

The findings are divided into two sections. The first section compares experiences of contact before and during the programme to examine if this increased contact helped improve father–child relationships. The second section explores whether these additional opportunities for contact facilitated the acquisition of the parenting skills fathers were being taught while on the programme.

Families' experiences of contact before and during the programme

Regardless of whether the father had been on remand or sentenced, families reported a noticeable difference in the amount and quality of contact they experienced once they joined the Families Matter programme. Prior to taking part in the programme, limited telephone contact was reported. Staff shortages had resulted in an unpredictable prison regime, with fathers' access to telephones frequently being curtailed with little advance warning. This meant that fathers were unable to contact their families as expected, frequently leaving children and partners feeling angry, annoyed, fearful, hurt and/or worried about their fathers. This was believed to damage children's wellbeing (as well as the wellbeing of fathers and partners) and to contribute to more negative communicative patterns within the family. It also meant that conversations were often cut short due to the number of people seeking to use the telephone in a short amount of time:

> You get to use the phone at night for five minutes and you are locked back up again, so your mental state isn't good at all. [...] Then when you phone the wife [...] you would be in a bad mood. [...] It is not good for the kids. [...] When they don't get that [phone call] it makes them sad. And then it makes you sad. [...] It is a vicious circle. (Participant 9 – Father)

Concerns were also expressed about the normal prison visits. Some family members reported feeling judged while attending these visits, damping their desire to continue visitation and contributing to negative feelings towards fathers/partners for exposing them to these situations:

> The [normal prison] visits [...] were stressful, very short, very upsetting. [...] Just feeling judged as a parent with a new child going into a prison. [...] Sometimes I would have felt angry like, because of what you are going through [...] and a bit frustrated maybe, with [father]. (Participant 42 – Family member)

Fathers and family members described how prison security protocols, designed to prevent the passing of contraband, restricted the ability of fathers to move and interact with their children, inhibiting natural father–child interactions:

> The wee 2 yr old was not going to sit on a seat for an hour. She gets up and starts wanting to toddle away. And if I stand up I get told to sit down. So I can't really play with her. [...] If I have to fix her wee skirt [...] straight away there is an officer standing behind me [...] they think I am trying to get something out of her clothes, or something. (Participant 8 – Father)

Parents were also worried about children witnessing aggressive incidents and/or being accidentally harmed by prison staff as they sought to intervene to prevent the smuggling of contraband or inappropriate behaviour during normal prison visits:

> On the normal visit [...] they [another couple] were fighting in the middle of the visit and [...] he had punched a woman in the face and [...] luckily enough it was the two wee ones [children], and we were able to keep their heads away and they didn't really notice what was going on. Like if it had been the two bigger ones [children] [...] it would have been terrible. They wouldn't have went back in [to the prison]. (Participant 36 – Family member)

> It just worries you that something is going to kick off [...] and before you know it the prison officers are in and [...] they don't think of a child [...] seeing this and what it may do to them. They are only there to solve a problem. (Participant 4 – Father)

While fathers and partners understood the need for prison staff to act quickly to intervene in situations, they were worried about the potential impact witnessing these events may have on their children:

> Them [normal prison] visits [...] there's been a few people jumped on [...] who were bringing in contraband. [...] It had a big impact on the kids. My wee girl started crying, thinking that that was the way I was being treated. And the missus too. (Participant 9 – Father)

> We have seen stuff that I would never have wanted them [children] to see, but what do you do? (Participant 37 – Family member)

The amount of people attending the normal prison visits also meant that these were often very noisy. This was perceived as adding to the stressful nature of the visit, as well as being challenging for children with autism or other developmental disorders:

> It was that loud [...] you couldn't hear yourself think, let alone hear what you were saying. So we argued quite a bit. [...] He [father] couldn't hear me and then I was getting frustrated. [...] It's stressful. (Participant 41 – Family member)

> My son can't handle noise, so when he comes up and visits, he [...] is basically punishing himself [...] because he does suffer from ADHD in a way that noise really does affect his

way of thinking. And I can see him putting his hands over his ears, and it hurts me to watch him. But he doesn't want to miss the visit so he puts himself through this. (Participant 12 – Father)

In some cases, fathers explained that they had to coax their children to attend the normal prison visits due to their child's dislike of the noise:

She has said to me a few times "Daddy I don't want to go to them wee [normal] visits again because they are too noisy". But I end up coaxing her and saying "I have loads of sweeties love, for you". (Participant 17 – Father)

In contrast, the family friendly visits provided by the Families Matter programme were viewed as being less stressful and offering a more normalised environment for father–child interactions:

I think it is a bit of normality for the kids […] as normal as it can be. […] They just really loved it. Getting to eat lunch together, just having [father] able to play with them and talk to them and if one of them needed one on one attention he [father] was able to do that and […] it was excellent (Participant 36 – Family member)

The family visits differed substantially from the normal prison visits, both in their duration (four hours compared to one hour) and in how fathers were able to interact with their children. Unlike the normal prison visits, fathers were not restricted in their movements so they could play, run, walk and eat with their children. Prison staff overseeing the special family visits were also mindful of how their actions could be interpreted by children and, while security concerns remained important, they were balanced with the needs of children and families:

He [father] can get up and interact with them [children]. […] That was the main difference. […] It is a whole lot more relaxed. Yes, you are being watched but you are […] not feeling as if you were stepping out of line if you move one way or […] another way. (Participant 36 -Family member)

The less stressful nature of these family visits was perceived as being particularly beneficial for children:

The family visits were, yeah. I would rather have them than the other [normal] visits. […] It was more relaxing and we looked forward to that one instead of the normal one. […] It was better for the children and it was a lot less stressful for everyone. (Participant 41 – Family members)

As such, the family visits were viewed as providing more quality father–child contact, providing fathers with an opportunity to rebuild/strengthen relationships with their children:

It has just built that bond back, because he [father] was losing it with [child]. […] Whenever he went inside [to prison] […] it was like [child] thought [father] had just left him. […] He hated [father] and resented him. So […] with the [family] visits they regained it again. (Participant 41 – Family member)

The Families Matter programme also sought to increase family contact by providing extra telephone access to fathers at times which were convenient for families. The residential nature of the programme facilitated this increased telephone access and through speaking with their children on the telephone, it was argued that fathers could continue to parent their children from prison. Fathers and families believed this telephone contact was a very important mechanism by which fathers could maintain contact with their children in between visits:

> You can just jump on the phone whenever you feel like it. [...] It definitely is [very important] like. (Participant 10 – Father)

Families responded very positively to the additional opportunities for family contact provided by the Families Matter programme. Accounts of children becoming happier, acting out less, relationships improving and fathers becoming more attuned to the needs of children were frequently heard:

> It did improve [relationships with children] because [...] they [children] were happier. It lifted their wee spirits [...] it was like, just like they had him again. (Participant 40 -Family member)

> Yes, we are a lot more happy. A lot more positive. [...] [Without the Families Matter programme] maybe we wouldn't be together. Wouldn't be as close. Because them one hour [normal] visits are horrendous. [...] We could have drifted. [...] Because they [normal visits] are so stressful, the one hour visits, you sort of think, you know, you go down there, by the time you get in there, the noise, he [father] is not allowed off the seat, he can't bond with the child, all the stress. [...] You know, I mightn't have went up every week. The family visit like nearly made you go up. (Participant 40 – Family member)

However, while these family visits provided a less stressful environment for family interactions and helped to prevent family relationships deteriorating, improvements in the quality of family interactions were predominately attributed to the new parenting skills fathers were acquiring as part of the programme. They believed that these skills helped fathers to better identify and meet children's needs and fathers were frequently witnessed using these skills during the special family visits and on the telephones to improve their relationships with their children:

> Before, I thought I was a brilliant father [...] But these courses [...] you can maybe identify if things are wrong with them [children] more than I used to [...] you are able to communicate better with them and try to identify what's wrong. [...] It has given me a better bond with them [...] it has given me more confidence. (Participant 3 – Father)

The role of contact in skill acquisition

Both fathers and staff agreed that it was essential that fathers had an opportunity to put into practice the parenting skills they were acquiring during the programme, if these skills were to become embedded:

> Theory is a great thing [...] we all need to do theory, but you know there is nothing like a bit of practical. (Participant 12 – Father)

Staff explained that when designing the Families Matter programme, they had deliberately sought to increase the quality and quantity of family contact available so as to improve family relationships and allow fathers to practise their newly acquired parenting skills. Fathers were actively encouraged by staff to use their new skills during telephone conservations and visits with their children. As part of the programme, staff delivering the parenting classes were also present during the special family visits to support fathers as they used these new skills in their interactions with their children. Staff were witnessed monitoring and supporting fathers as they attempted to put these skills into practice. In this way, staff were able to observe father–child relationships, assist when required and provide personalised feedback on fathers' use of these skills:

> They put it [newly acquired parenting skills] into practice on the [family] visits and [...] we will be looking out to make sure [...] that they are getting down to their child's eye level to speak to them. Down on the floor and playing with them. (Participant 30 – Staff)

> Everybody is doing this course obviously to learn and to put in practice what they have learned through the classes at that family visit. (Participant 3 – Father)

Fathers explained that having the opportunity to rehearse new parenting skills was facilitating their acquisition and consolidation of these skills. Using these skills also built up their confidence in their parenting abilities and gave them additional tools to use to improve their relationships with their children:

> I've learned a good wee bit from it [Families Matter programme] [...] how to discipline them [children] and [...] I've been trying it out at the [family] visits and it has been working. [...] My wee lad started to mess about and [I] got on the floor [...] got down to his level and said "[name] get up on my knee now". And he done it like that there. And [...] his ma was sitting telling him to get up and he wouldn't do it. [...] I was actually a wee bit shocked [that it worked]! (Participant 10 – Father)

> You know what teenagers are like. When you phone them they say hello and it's hard to get conversation out of them. But you learn things in them [parenting] classes to say to your kids to get a conversation out of them. [...] That helps. (Participant 7 – Father)

Family members reported noticing fathers using their newly acquired parenting skills in their interactions with their children and were impressed with the effect this was having on their family relationships. In particular, accounts of fathers speaking to their children for longer periods of time and more often on the telephone were frequently heard, as well as fathers being able to interact better with their children:

> The best thing about the four hour [family] visit, whatever [father] had learned in the Families Matter programme, he was able to put it into practice [...] which was really exciting for him and for her [daughter]. [...] It was really good because it let me see that I could trust [father] with [daughter] [...] I knew he would be OK, he would be able to cope (Participant 42 – Family member)

> She [partner] has noticed a change in me [father]. [...] Like I would ask more about the kids. I would ask him [child] on the phone, I would talk more and ask what was he doing at school, how was he getting on, what have you done, have you been good? You know things like that. (Participant 10 – Father)

Many fathers believed that they would be able to continue to use these newly acquired parenting skills on their release from prison, as they felt the opportunities available to rehearse these skills during the programme had been sufficient to fully internalise and assimilate them:

> At the end of the day, I am learning stuff which I never knew I could have done before, that I'll be able to practise outside [...] with my kids, emotions and self-esteem and stuff. (Participant 3 – Father)

Only one father was more cautious in this respect, arguing that while the opportunities for increased contact during the programme had been very beneficial, as fathers continued to be imprisoned they would remain limited in their ability to fully internalise these skills until they returned home to their families and were using these skills on a more frequent basis:

> I [have] learned from the parenting class [...] passive, assertive and aggressive [parenting styles], and stuff like that. There was a couple of other things too [...] but you are in jail. [...] You need to be in a home environment to put anything into practice that you learn. (Participant 15 – Father)

Unless fathers were being released immediately on completion of the Families Matter programme, both fathers on remand and sentenced were worried about how the improvements in their father–child relationships would be maintained beyond the completion of the programme. As families could only avail themselves of the additional telephone contact and family visits during the Families Matter programme, fathers and their families were concerned about how a return to pre-programme levels of contact would affect their father–child relationships:

> It is good for the child but it is bad at the end [of the programme] because [...] now he [child] is asking [...] "Is it the normal one [visit] or is it the family one [visit]?" Because if it is not that [family visit] one, he doesn't want to go. (Participant 41 – Family member)

> You have a child where [...] [on the family visits] you can run over and grab her [...] play, do the things that mothers and fathers should be doing. [...] And then the next thing is [...] [you go back to the normal visits and] Daddy can't move. [...] Daddy's not allowed off this pink chair. [...] The child doesn't see the bigger picture, they think that their Daddy doesn't care about them anymore. Their Daddy doesn't want them [...] so you can actually give a child a complex. (Participant 12 – Father)

Given the restrictions on movement and physical contact fathers experienced during the normal prison visits, as well as the uncertainties over telephone access prior to their participation in the Families Matter programme, it seemed that fathers were going to struggle to use their new parenting skills once the programme ended. As improvements in father–child relationships were generally attributed to fathers' use of these parenting skills, it seemed very likely that these improvements would be undone if regular, quality contact in which fathers could use and rehearse their parenting skills was not provided beyond the completion of the programme. Accordingly, the lack of a plan for how to sustain and progress the benefits obtained from participating in the Families Matter programme beyond its completion until the fathers' release from prison may undermine its potential long-term effectiveness.

Discussion

Based on these findings, families responded very positively to the increased contact available as part of the Families Matter programme. The additional telephone access and provision of special family visits was attributed to not only increasing the amount of contact between fathers and their children but also the quality of this contact, providing more opportunities for deep and meaningful father–child interactions to occur than were ordinarily available within the prison. Fathers were also provided with opportunities to put their newly acquired parenting skills into practice, allowing fathers to master the application of these skills and use them to improve their relationships with their children.

These findings, therefore, indicate that prison based parenting programmes should ensure that opportunities to engage in deep and meaningful interactions with children and to use the parenting skills being taught are provided, if relationships between imprisoned parents and their children are to be improved.

The extent to which prison based parenting programmes may need to provide additional opportunities for contact to facilitate this type of parent–child interaction will vary depending on the opportunities for contact routinely available within a prison, the experience of families accessing these opportunities and the length of the father's imprisonment. Policies, practices and procedures surrounding prison visitation, telephone usage and letter writing vary substantially between different jurisdictions and even within different prisons within the same jurisdiction (Besemer et al., 2011; Hutton, 2016; Murray et al., 2007; Sharratt, 2014). As a result, the quantity and quality of father–child contact will differ from prison to prison, depending on the regime in that prison and its security status, influencing the opportunities fathers have to rehearse their parenting skills and use these skills to improve father–child relationships. Consequently, when establishing a prison based parenting programme, careful consideration should be given to the existing opportunities for family contact to assess if these opportunities are sufficient for mastering the parenting skills being taught on the programme, facilitate quality father–child interactions and cope with the length of time fathers are imprisoned for.

Within Maghaberry Prison, fathers' and family members' experiences of family contact prior to the Families Matter programme highlighted the importance of providing additional opportunities for increased contact to facilitate parenting skill acquisition and improvements in father–child relationships. As Maghaberry Prison is a high security adult male prison, it is unsurprising that it may adopt stricter, more security focused protocols surrounding family contact than may be present in other prisons. The continuing detention of political prisoners within Maghaberry Prison also amplified this focus on security (CJINI, 2015). For this reason, the additional opportunities for family engagement provided on the Families Matter programme were key to its success, as the opportunities for family contact ordinarily available within the prison limited the acquisition of the parenting skills being taught on the programme or the use of these skills in father–child interactions. This additional family contact, therefore, helped prevent a deterioration in family relationships, facilitated the acquisition of parenting skills and provided fathers with an opportunity to use these skills to improve their father–child relationships.

Of course, the provision of such additional opportunities for contact may not be as necessary in prisons which already adopt longer, less restrictive, child friendly visiting practices. For example, in Sweden, it has been argued that the more frequent use of private family visits, open prisons, home leave, telephone and written communications have protected children from some of the negative effects of parental imprisonment (Murray et al., 2007). Similarly, in the Netherlands, more humane prison conditions and a tendency to provide more opportunities for family contact has been credited with helping to reduce some of the negative effects of parental imprisonment (Besemer et al., 2011). For this reason, whether a prison based parenting programme will benefit from including additional opportunities for family contact, will depend on the quality and quantity of family contact ordinarily available within that prison.

However, even if additional opportunities for family contact are provided, the extent to which improvements to father–child relationships are maintained and parenting skills retained in the longer-term is questionable, if there is a lack of a strategic vision for how this work will be progressed if fathers continue to be imprisoned beyond the completion of the programme. Similar to previous research, the findings indicate that prison visits which impose restrictions on movement and contact can limit the extent to which fathers can engage in deep and meaningful interactions with children and improve strained father–child relationships (Dennison et al., 2017; Hutton, 2016; Sharratt, 2014). According to Sharratt (2014), the quality of parent–child relationships prior to imprisonment can significantly affect children's motivation to maintain contact with their imprisoned parent. For those with positive relationships, children are believed to be motivated to maintain contact, despite the stresses and challenges they may encounter while doing so (Sharratt, 2014). Nevertheless, these children require regular contact if their wellbeing and positive father–child relationships are to be sustained (Sharratt, 2014). The additional telephone access and extra family visits available on the Families Matter programme played an important part in facilitating regular deep and meaningful contact between such children and their fathers. In contrast, for those with strained relationships, children are believed to be less willing to maintain contact and it is hypothesised that being exposed to stress or challenges may further decrease their motivation to maintain contact, potentially leading to relationship breakdown (Sharratt, 2014). Sharratt (2014) argues that under the right conditions such relationships can be improved. The findings from this research suggest that enhancing the fathers' parenting skills and allowing them to use these skills in the context of the less stressful and restrictive family friendly visits helped fathers to rebuild strained father–child relationships. However, a return to pre-programme levels of contact could threaten these newly rebuilt relationships, as children and fathers revert back to contact conditions which restricted meaningful interactions. In such circumstances, improvements to father–child relations may be undone and relationships may again begin to deteriorate.

Moreover, returning to pre-programme levels of contact would inhibit the ability of fathers to rehearse and use the parenting skills they had acquired. When teaching new parenting skills, skill maintenance is a key component of skill acquisition (Lindhiem, Higa, Trentacosta, Herschell, & Kolko, 2014). Fathers need to be able to continue to use their parenting skills throughout the remainder of their imprisonment if they are to retain these skills. Returning to pre-programme levels of contact was going to immediately inhibit the ability of fathers to use some of these skills due to the prison's policy of restricting movement and physical contact during normal prison visitation. One possible solution was to only allow those nearly at the end of their imprisonment to complete the programme but, by this time, family relationships may have broken down beyond repair. For this reason, fathers at any stage of their imprisonment were eligible to participate in the Families Matter programme but this meant there was a need to ensure that fathers remained able to practise their skills and maintain their family relationship during the remainder of their imprisonment until their release. Families Matter programme staff were aware of this issue and were seeking to remedy it but were restricted in their ability to do so without wider changes in the prison policies, procedures and practices surrounding family contact. Accordingly, despite the prison investing in a programme designed to improve parenting skills and family relationships, the potential long-term effectiveness of the programme was limited by the lack of a clear vision for how this work should be progressed and the prison's own policies, practices and procedures surrounding family contact.

There are, however, a number of limitations which must be borne in mind when interpreting the findings of this research. In particular, its sample size and focus on one parenting programme restricts the generalisability of its findings. Further, the lack of a follow-up limits the ability of the study to assess how a return to pre-programme levels of contact affected parenting skills retention or father–child relationships in the long term. Future research should seek to overcome these limitations as well as identify how variations in prison policies, procedures and practices may affect the long-term effectiveness of prison based parenting programmes.

Nevertheless, despite these limitations, this research offers a number of insights into how prisons can enhance family contact and strengthen prison based parenting programmes to improve outcomes for children. First, prison based parenting programmes should ensure that imprisoned parents have an opportunity to rehearse the skills they are acquiring, if they are to master the performance of these skills, use these skills to improve father–child relationships and minimise the negative impact of parental imprisonment on children. If suitable opportunities for family contact are not regularly available within a prison, the provision of such opportunities will be important for the potential success of prison based parenting programmes and their ability to improve child outcomes and family relationships.

Secondly, there needs to be clear plans for how the gains made as a result of participation in prison based parenting programmes will be maintained beyond programme completion until release, with different plans in place to cope with long term and short term imprisonment. If opportunities to maintain family contact and rehearse parenting skills are restricted upon programme completion, father–child relationships may begin to deteriorate and newly acquired parenting skills may be lost. This is particularly an issue in prisons whereby policies, practices and procedures surrounding visitation, telephone access and letter-writing may be more restrictive and not conducive to quality father–child interactions. In such situations, these policies, practices and procedures may ultimately undermine efforts to strengthen family relationships and weaken the long-term effectiveness of such programmes. Undermining family relationships can not only result in adverse outcomes for children but also hinder attempts to reduce re-offending, reintegration and desistance for fathers on their release from prison (Brunton-Smith & McCarthy, 2016; Duwe & Clark, 2013; Mears, Cochran, Siennick, & Bales, 2012; Samposn & Laub, 1993; Visher & Travis, 2003).

Thirdly, depending on the prison, it may be necessary to review the policies, practice and procedures surrounding normal prison visitation so that security concerns can be better balanced with the needs of children. In particular, this research highlighted parents' worries about the potential for children to witness aggressive incidents during normal visitation by both those participating in visits and prison staff. Some steps that can be taken to address these concerns include moving towards a model of visitation which facilitates private visits, greater use of home leave, more child-friendly family visiting arrangements, the provision of family visiting slots (in which individuals are carefully chosen because of their reduced likelihood of engaging in conflict) and providing additional staff training on how to respond to conflict situations in the presence of children. The research also suggests that the suitability of normal prison visitation for those with autism and/or other developmental disorders may need to be reviewed to ensure that these children are not being disadvantaged, due to the failure of the prison to consider their particular needs.

Lastly, prison policies regarding telephone access may need to be revised so that regular contact between parents and their children can be maintained during imprisonment. In particular, sufficient telephones should be available to meet the needs of those imprisoned, imprisoned parents should have access to telephones at times convenient to families so children can speak to their imprisoned parent and making a telephone call should not be so costly that it hinders rather than facilitates frequent contact.

Accordingly, while prison based parenting programmes can improve parenting skills and father–child relationships, their potential long-term effectiveness may be restricted by prison policies, practices and procedures which inhibit the maintenance of these gains throughout the remainder of the parent's imprisonment. A failure to consider this issue may result in parenting skills being lost and improvements in father–child relationships being undone, contributing to relationship breakdown and adverse outcomes for children. In developing justice policies, policymakers should, therefore, pay more attention to how prison policies, practices and procedures may have unintended knock-on consequences for the wellbeing of children and their outcomes, as well as reducing offending.

Disclosure statement

No potential conflict of interest was reported by the authors.

Funding

This work was supported by Barnardo's Northern Ireland under Grant number R2173SSP.

ORCID

David Hayes ⓘ http://orcid.org/0000-0001-7053-9069
Michelle Butler ⓘ http://orcid.org/0000-0002-6983-6215
John Devaney ⓘ http://orcid.org/0000-0001-8300-8339
Andrew Percy ⓘ http://orcid.org/0000-0003-4156-1536

References

Andrews, D., & Dowden, C. (2005). Managing correctional treatment for reduced recidivism: A meta-analytic review of programme integrity. *Legal and Criminological Psychology, 10*, 173–187. doi:10.1348/135532505X36723

Barnardo's. (2015). *The evaluation of the community support for offenders' families service*. Ilford: Barnardo's.

Barr, R., Brito, N., Zocca, J., Reina, S., Rodriguez, J., & Shauffer, C. (2011). The baby elmo program: Improving teen father-child interactions within juvenile justice facilities. *Children and Youth Services Review, 33*(9), 1555–1562. doi:10.1016/j.childyouth.2011.03.020

Barr, R., Morin, M., Brito, N., Richeda, B., Rodriguez, J., & Shauffer, C. (2014). Delivering services to incarcerated teen fathers: A pilot intervention to increase the quality of father-infant interactions during visitation. *Psychological Services, 11*(1), 10–21. doi:10.1037/a0034877

Besemer, S., van der Geest, V., Murray, J., Bijleveld, C. C. J. H., & Farrington, D. P. (2011). The relationship between parental imprisonment and offspring offending in England and the Netherlands. *British Journal of Criminology, 51*(2), 413–437. doi:10.1093/bjc/azq072

Boswell, G., Poland, F., & Price, A. (2010). *Prison based family support: An evaluation of the effectiveness f the family support worker role piloted in four English prisons during 2009–10*. London: Ministry of Justice National Offender Management Service.

Braun, V., & Clarke, V. (2006). Using thematic analysis in psychology. *Qualitative Research in Psychology, 3*(2), 77–101.

Bronte-Tinkew, J., Carrano, J., Allen, T., Bowie, L., Mbawa, K., & Matthews, G. (2008). *Elements of promising practice for fatherhood programs: Evidence-based research findings on programs for fathers*. Gaithersburg: U.S. Department of Health and Human Services Office of Family Assistance.

Brunton-Smith, I., & McCarthy, D. J. (2016). The effects of prisoner attachment to family on re-entry outcomes: A longitudinal assessment. *British Journal of Criminology*, doi:10.1093/bjc/azv129

Bryman, A. (2008). *Social research methods*. Oxford: Oxford University Press.

Buston, K., Parkes, A., Thomson, H., Wight, D., & Fenton, C. (2012). Parenting interventions for male young offenders: A review of the evidence on what works. *Journal of Adolescence, 35*(3), 731–742. doi:10.1016/j.adolescence.2011.10.007

Butler, M. (2016). Prisoners and prison life. In D. Healy, C. Hamilton, Y. Daly, & M. Butler (Eds.), *The routledge handbook of Irish criminology* (pp. 337–355). Oxford: Taylor & Francis.

Butler, M., Hayes, D., Devaney, J., & Percy, A. (2015). *Strengthening family relations: Review of the families matter programme at maghaberry prison*. Belfast: Barnardo's NI.

Criminal Justice Inspection Northern Ireland. (2015). *Report of an unannounced inspection of Maghaberry prison 11–12 may 2015*. Belfast: Criminal Justice Inspection Northern Ireland.

Dennison, S., Smallbone, H., & Occhipinti, S. (2017). Understanding how incarceration challenges proximal processes in father-child relationships: Perspectives of imprisoned fathers. *Journal of Development Life Course Criminology, 3*(1), 15–38.

Duwe, G., & Clark, V. (2013). Blessed be the social tie that binds. *Criminal Justice Policy Review, 24*(3), 271–296. doi:10.1177/0887403411429724

Flynn, C., & Eriksson, A. (2015). *Children of prisoners*. Annandale: The Federation Press.

Foster, H., & Hagan, J. (2009). The mass incarceration of parents in America: Issues of race/ethnicity, collateral damage to children, and prisoner reentry. *Annals of the American Academy of Political and Social Science, 623*, 179–194. doi:10.1177/0002716208331123

Friedman, V. J., & Antal, A. B. (2005). Negotiating reality: A theory of action approach to intercultural competence. *Management Learning, 36*(1), 69–86. doi:10.1177/1350507605049904

Garland, D. (1990). *Punishment and modern society: A study in social theory*. Oxford: Clarendon Press.

Hagan, J., & Dinovitzer, R. (1999). Collateral consequences of imprisonment for children, communities, and prisoners. *Crime and Justice, 26*, 121–162. doi:10.1086/449296

Hagan, J., & Foster, H. (2012). Intergenerational educational effects of mass imprisonment in America. *Sociology of Education, 85*(3), 259–286. doi:10.1177/0038040711431587

Hoffmann, H. C., Byrd, A. L., & Kightlinger, A. M. (2010). Prison programs and services for incarcerated parents and their underage children: Results from a national survey of correctional facilities. *Prison Journal, 90*(4), 397–416. doi:10.1177/0032885510382087

Hollin, C. (1995). The meaning and implications of programme integrity. In J. Maguire (Ed.), *What works: Reducing reoffending – guidelines from research and practice* (pp. 193–206). Chichester: Wiley.

Hutton, M. (2016). Visiting time. *Probation Journal, 63*(3), 347–361. doi:10.1177/0264550516663644

Kim, J. W., Ritter, F. E., & Koubek, R. J. (2013). An integrated theory for improved skill acquisition and retention in the three stages of learning. *Theoretical Issues in Ergonomics Science, 14*(1), 22–37. doi:10.1080/1464536X.2011.573008

La Vigne, N. G., Naser, R. L., Brooks, L. E., & Castro, J. L. (2005). Examining the effect of incarceration and in-prison family contact on prisoners'family relationships. *Journal of Contemporary Criminal Justice, 21*(4), 314–335. doi:10.1177/1043986205281727

Lindhiem, O., Higa, J., Trentacosta, C. J., Herschell, A. D., & Kolko, D. J. (2014). Skill acquistion and utilization during evidence-based psychological treatments for childhood disruptive behavior problems: A review and meta-analysis. *Clinical Child and Family Psychological Review, 17*(1), 41–66.

Lipsey, M. W. (1995). What do we learn from 400 research studies on the effectiveness of treatment with juvenile delinquents. In J. Maguire (Ed.), *What works: Reducing reoffending: Guidelines from research and practice* (pp. 63–78). Chichester: Wiley.

Loper, A. B., & Tuerk, E. H. (2006). Parenting programs for incarcerated parents: Current research and future directions. *Criminal Justice Policy Review, 17*(4), 407–427. doi:10.1177/0887403406292692

McCrudden, E., Braiden, J. H., McCormack, P., Sloan, P., & Treacy, D. (2014). Stealing the smile from my child's face: A preliminary evaluation of the "being a dad" programme in a northern Ireland prison. *Child Care in Practice, 20*(3), 301–312.

Mears, D. P., Cochran, J. C., Siennick, S. E., & Bales, W. D. (2012). Prison visitation and recidivism. *Justice Quarterly, 29*(6), 888–918. doi:10.1080/07418825.2011.583932

Meek, R. (2007). Parenting education for young fathers in prison. *Child & Family Social Work, 12*(3), 239–247. doi:10.1111/j.1365-2206.2007.00456.x

Murray, J., Janson, C., & Farrington, D. P. (2007). Crime in adult offspring of prisoners – A cross-national comparison of two longitudinal samples. *Criminal Justice and Behavior, 34*(1), 133–149. doi:10.1177/009385806289549

Murray, J., & Murray, L. (2010). Parental incarceration, attachment and child psychopathology. *Attachment & Human Development, 12*(4), 289–309. doi:10.1080/14751790903416889

Newman, C., Fowler, C., & Cashin, A. (2011). The development of a parenting program for incarcerated mothers in Australia: A review of prison-based parenting programs. *Contemporary Nurse, 39*(1), 2–11.

Parson, T., Shils, E., & Smelser, N. (2001). *Toward a general theory of action: Theoretical foundations for the social sciences.* New Jersey: Transaction Publishers.

Poehlmann, J., Dallaire, D. H., Loper, A. B., & Shear, L. D. (2010). Children's contact with their incarcerated parents: Research findings and recommendations. *American Psychologist, 65*(6), 575–598.

Proctor, R. W., & Dutta, A. (1995). *Skill acquisition and human performance.* Thousand Oaks: Sage.

Purvis, M. (2013). Paternal incarceration and parenting programs in prison: A review paper. *Psychiatry Psychology and Law, 20*(1), 9–28. doi:10.1080/13218719.2011.615822

Samposn, R. J., & Laub, J. H. (1993). *Crime in the making: Pathways and turning points through life.* London: Cambridge University Press.

Sharratt, K. (2014). Children's experiences of contact with imprisoned parents: A comparison between four European countries. *European Journal of Criminology, 11*(6), 760–775. doi:10.1177/1477370814525936

Stokes, J. O., Jent, J. F., Weinstein, A., Davis, E. M., Brown, T. M., Cruz, L., & Wavering, H. (2016). Does practice make perfect? The relationship between self-reported treatment homework completion and parental skill acquisition and child behaviors. *Behavior Therapy*, *47*(4), 538–549. doi:10.1016/j.beth.2016.04.004

Visher, C., & Travis, J. (2003). Transitions from prison to community: Understanding individual pathways. *Annual Review of Sociology*, *29*, 89–113. doi:10.1146/annurev.soc.29.010202.095931

Wakefield, S., & Wildeman, C. (2011). Mass imprisonment and racial disparities in childhood behavioral problems. *Criminology & Public Policy*, *10*(3), 793–817. doi:10.1111/j.1745-9133. 2011.00740.x

Walmsley, R. (2016). *World prison population list* (11th ed.). London: Institute for Criminal Policy Research.

Wildeman, C. (2009). Parental imprisonment, the prison boom, and the concentration of childhood disadvantage. *Demography*, *46*(2), 265–280.

Wildeman, C. (2014). Parental incarceration, child homelessness, and the invisible consequences of mass imprisonment. *Annals of the American Academy of Political and Social Science*, *651*(1), 74–96. doi:10.1177/0002716213502921

Does Fatherhood Training in Prison Improve Fathering Skills and Reduce Family Challenges?

Gunnar Vold Hansen

ABSTRACT

The Norwegian Correctional Service offers a program called "Fathers in Prison", aimed at helping incarcerated fathers to have better contact with their children during their sentence and after release. On the basis of 38 semi-structured interviews with prisoners who have completed the program, we would argue that there is reason to believe that the program enhances the participants' fathering skills. Feedback from the participants showed that "Fathers in Prison" helps fathers take greater responsibility for their children's situation, their fathering skills improve and father–child contact is enhanced. However, the program appears to have little influence on the situation of the prisoner's family while he is still imprisoned. There is no indication that participation by the father in the program implies better support for his children and family than they would otherwise receive. The conclusion is consequently that the program helps participants to function better as fathers both during and after imprisonment, but that it does not reduce challenges in prisoners' families to any great extent.

Penal policy in Norway is based on a humanistic approach. In Parliamentary Report No. 37 (2007–2008). "Punishment that works—less crime—a safer society", the Government strongly emphasized that punishment should be more than just locking up offenders. A sentence must contain elements that enhance the likelihood that the offender will live a life without crime upon release. It is strongly emphasized that the prison sentence should prepare offenders for their release and transition back into the community. Offenders lose their freedom when serving time, but do not lose their rights to public services. The rights to health and social services that the individual had before the sentence will not be lost during imprisonment.

Preparation for release is done in various ways, including cooperation with employment and education services in order to provide opportunities for prisoners to study and gain qualifications during their time in prison (Hansen, 2017). During the sentence, the correctional services may offer various types of courses, or programs as they are commonly called. Many of these programs aim to motivate convicts to change their ways to prepare them better for a life of freedom.

If the offender identifies with other roles, such as that of a father, this can make him more determined to distance himself from the role of a criminal (Lösel, Pugh, Markson, Souza, & Lanskey, 2012). Activities that help prisoners to see themselves in a new role can thus motivate them to desist from criminal activity (Ronel & Segev, 2014). In order to get the convicts to identify themselves more as a father than a criminal, the correctional service has developed a program entitled "Fathers in Prison". A previous article has shown that participants in this program became more concerned with their role as a father and felt that it conflicted with criminal activity. The program therefore appeared to fulfill its main purpose (Hansen, 2017).

The family will also be affected when someone is sent to prison, and for children such a situation may be problematic. An important goal for the Norwegian correctional service is to reduce the negative consequences of imprisonment for the inmates' relatives (Parliamentary White Paper No. 37, 2007–2008). The correctional services have a duty to identify the needs offenders may have during and after the prison sentence. If the individual agrees, the correctional services will use the information obtained to contact relevant health and social services to meet his or her needs both during and after imprisonment (Hansen & Samuelsen, 2016). Such an obligation does not exist in relation to the relatives. However, a program such as "Fathers in Prison" may also be an opportunity to take care of the convicts' families. The main question raised in this article is therefore: Does the "Fathers in Prison" program improve prisoners' fathering skills and limit the negative impact of the imprisonment on their families? The article is based on a re-analysis of data collected in connection with the evaluation of the program (Hansen, Arvesen, & Tonholm, 2013).

Background

As early as 1965, the first systematic study of prisoners' families was published (Morris, 1965). In 1983, a study concluded that challenges with regard to income, work and responsibility for the children created major problems for the spouse—in practice, the mother—who was not imprisoned (Ferraro, Johnson, Jorgensen, & Bolton, 1983). The term "forgotten victims", referring to children of inmates, began to be used in the same year (Matthews, 1983). The fact that prisoners also realized that they had a role as a father and husband to relate to after release was revealed in a survey from 1989. This survey showed that, in spite of being prisoners, they saw themselves as active fathers in the future and wanted to improve their fathering skills (Hairston, 1989).

Children tend to respond in different ways to the imprisonment of their father. Some find it a relief that the father goes to prison; this often applies in families with high levels of alcohol/drug abuse and violence (Poehlmann, Dallaire, Loper, & Shear, 2010). We also know that some children find it satisfactory that their dad is in prison because then they know where he is and they do not have to be afraid of him in the same way as if he goes off somewhere while he is out (Grambo, 2000). However, for most children, the imprisonment of a father or mother is a traumatic experience (Boswell, 2002; Egge, 2004). Many parents tell their children little about what is happening, which makes the children uneasy. Some children have difficulty relating to an event they do not understand. The adults' silence can be problematic in such situations, and some children are afraid that they are to blame for their father's absence.

Unfortunately, it is not only the relationship with the father which is affected by imprisonment. It also affects children's relationships with those around them. In some cases, prisoners' children who are open about the imprisonment have reported positive reactions from e.g. their school, both from teachers and fellow students (Boswell, 2002; Egge, 2004). There are also examples of children of prisoners meeting each other and finding it helpful to discuss their experiences with others in the same situation. However, one survey showed that two-thirds of these children reported that they were sad. Furthermore, 16% of them said they suffered from anxiety as a result of their father being in prison (Hamsund & Sandvik, 2010). They are subjected to more bullying than other children and they grow up in homes with greater financial problems than most. They therefore have poorer living conditions than other children and a higher incidence of social and mental problems (Smith, Grimshaw, Romeo, & Knapp, 2007). We also find that children of prisoners have greater learning difficulties than other children and are more likely to develop behavioral problems and turn to crime themselves (Boswell, 2002; Farrington, 2005). Figures from Norway show that 24% of inmates have a father who has been in prison (Friestad & Skog Hansen, 2004).

A comprehensive meta-analysis of how the imprisonment of fathers affects their children shows a clear correlation between the father's imprisonment and the children's behavioral problems (Murray, Farrington, & Sekol, 2012). In a review article, Christmann, Turliuc, and Mairean (2012) conclude that there is strong and comprehensive evidence that children of inmates have a greater incidence of mental illness than others. A comprehensive European study has also documented the relationship between the father's imprisonment and the children's mental ill health (Jones et al., 2013).

It is normally important for children to find that they can still have contact with their father after his incarceration. More letters between children and parents in prison meant less depression and somatic disorders in the children (Dallaire, Ciccone, & Wilson, 2010). Good contact between father and children during the sentence also has consequences for the post-release situation. It has been shown that better contact (visits and letters) during imprisonment also improved contact after release (Poehlmann et al., 2010). We also see that children who have contact with their imprisoned father report less alienation from the father after release (Shlafer & Poehlmann, 2010).

A program for fathers

The quality of contact between father and children is not only dependent on how the correctional services facilitate the contact but also on the ability of the father to take on a parental role. Many inmates have had their own fathers in prison, been in child care and had other childhood experiences which have led to a lack of good role models to teach them fathering. The correctional services in a number of countries have therefore offered imprisoned fathers various training programs to help them become as good fathers as possible (Hunter, Skrine, Turnbull, Kazimirski, & Pritchard, 2013). Some of these courses for inmates have been regular parenting courses aimed at families outside prison, while others have been training programs developed specifically for correctional purposes (Hoffmann, Byrd, & Kightlinger, 2010; Loper & Tuerk, 2006). Improving the ability of the fathers to help their children, during their sentence and especially afterwards, can be an important strategy for reducing the challenges of children of prisoners. In a review article, Purvis (2013) points out that only a small percentage of fatherhood programs have been evaluated. However, she concludes that such programs should have two objectives. Firstly, they should enhance the quality of father–child interaction. Secondly, they should help to reduce the risk of the children also becoming criminals. The question posed by the present article is therefore: "Does fatherhood training in prison improve fathering skills and reduce family challenges?"

"Fathers in Prison"

In Norway, the correctional services have developed a program for incarcerated fathers called "Fathers in Prison". The program was developed in a Norwegian prison in the years 2004–2005, inspired by a similar Scottish program. Since then, it has been adjusted several times, partly on the basis of the experience of the instructors and the feedback they have received from the participants. The main aim of the program is to help offenders gain new perspectives on their criminal behavior and how this affects their children and other family members. The program is thus intended to motivate inmates to take responsibility for living a life in accordance with the rules of society. By participating in the program, prisoners will enhance their knowledge, skills and attitudes to better enable them to perform fatherhood in accordance with the expectations of their children, family members and society at large. Key elements of the program are (Hansen et al., 2013):

- Network map, family and family situation
- Communication
- Developmental theory—child development
- Role theory—roles and role models
- Emotions—how to relate to emotions—coping
- Challenges and problem solving
- Child health—prevention and treatment
- Children's rights—parents' responsibilities
- Public services—who can we cooperate with?

All potential participants are interviewed before the start of the program and only motivated inmates considered likely to benefit from the program are invited to participate. Sexual offenders or others considered unsuitable are not invited. In order to motivate participants to begin a change process, the course is dialogue-based and the instructors employ principles from theories of motivational interviewing (Rollnick & Miller, 1995) and the so-called "wheel of change" (Prochaska & DiClemente, 1982) in communication with the participants. The program also includes learner-based activities, such as making a DVD movie where participants show their family how they live and what life is like in prison. The program also requires participants to plan and implement a family day. The entire program takes four weeks and consists of 16 sessions, four per week. The program is led by two instructors, who have received special training and authorization.

The participants in this program indicated that they had become more responsible, gave more thought to how their crimes affected others, learned how to be more involved with their children and communicate better with close family members, and realized that they ought to stop their criminal activity. They also found it important that the program was an arena for support by the other participants and the instructors in such a change process (Hansen, 2017).

A number of Norwegian prisons now include family quarters within the prison compound where the offender can stay with his family for short periods (usually 24–48 hours) during his sentence. It is generally a requirement that he has completed a "Fathers in Prison" program before being allowed to use this family house. The program is therefore an important part of the correctional strategy to improve contact between the inmate and his children.

Data collection and method

We wished to obtain maximum insight into how the participants experienced the program, and therefore chose to interview all participants (Danermark, Ekström, Jacobsen, & Karlsson, 2003). Data collection was conducted in three prisons in eastern Norway. These were the only three prisons that planned to implement the program during the six months we had set aside for data collection. Two of these were closed high-security prisons and one was an open prison. The study was approved by the Privacy Ombudsman for Research and was conducted in accordance with the relevant regulations. These state that study participation must be voluntary and that data must be stored on password-protected computers in secure networks. All course participants in the three prisons agreed to participate in the study and were informed orally and in writing that they could withdraw from the study at any time.

All participants in the three prisons were to be interviewed three times—at the beginning of the program, immediately after conclusion of the program and about six months later. For various reasons such as release and transfer to other prisons, the number of participants interviewed decreased from 16 (one prison had six participants and the other two had five) in the first round to 13 in the second round and nine in the final round of interviews. A total of 38 interviews were conducted. The interviews took place in the prisons in a designated room where we could sit undisturbed with each participant. At the two high-security prisons, the interviewer, like any other visitor, was equipped with an alarm, but this was not practiced in the open prison. The interviews lasted between 20 minutes and one hour, depending on what the participant wanted to talk about.

The participants had a wide variety of backgrounds. Their ages ranged from the early twenties to well into their forties. They all had children; some only one child, others more than one. Some had young children, while others had children in their teens. Some were in a stable marriage or cohabitation, while others had had children with more than one woman and had more than one ex-partner/ex-wife. Sometimes the inmate's family lived near the prison, in other cases the family lived at some distance from the prison, even abroad. Some participants had recently begun their sentence, while others were nearing the end. The length of the sentences also varied considerably.

The interview guide was semi-structured, enabling us to emphasize an open dialogue with the interviewees and allow them as far as possible to direct the conversation (Kvale, 2001). The interview guide was therefore primarily used as a checklist to ensure that we had covered all the planned topics. The same researcher interviewed the participants on all three occasions. This meant that the researcher and participant got to know each other quite well and the conversation flowed fairly easily in most cases.

All interviews were recorded digitally. A number of participants agreed to the interview and the recording on condition that the interview would only be available to the interviewer and that personal information and reactions would be treated with care. We considered it important to respect this request. The three researchers who conducted the interviews therefore studied their recordings separately, and only transcribed the parts that were considered to be of central importance. The separate analyses were made directly on the basis of the audio files, where we noted down meaning condensation for each statement. These meaning condensations were then categorized (Kvale, 2001). Afterwards, each researcher presented an analysis of his/her own data to the two others, explaining how the interviews were processed and which meaning condensations and categorizations were made. Interviews were initially analyzed on the basis of Malterud's systematic text condensation (Malterud, 2012) where we followed her procedure through the four steps she describes: (1) total impression—from chaos to themes; (2) identifying and sorting meaning units—from themes to codes; (3) condensation—from code to meaning; (4) synthesizing—from condensation to descriptions and concepts.

We emphasized respect for the informants' privacy, and some of the quotations presented here have therefore been adjusted in order to conceal their identity. For the same reason, we also decided not to provide information on the participants' background.

There have been no interviews of the participants' children. There are several reasons for that. Some were practical challenges; like that the children lived some distance away from the prisons. The main reason, however, was the consideration of the children themselves. A number of surveys have shown that children of inmates perceive the situation as traumatic (Boswell, 2002; Egge, 2004). We were afraid of that interviewing the children could enhance such trauma. We therefore decided not to interview any children.

Presentation of the data

Attitude change

All participants had volunteered for the program. This indicates that they were basically all interested in their family and their role as a father, but in addition several participants emphasized that the program had made them realize that they had had the wrong priorities in their lives so far.

> I wasn't so much there for them before. I used to think about lots of other stuff, but the most important thing is the people around you. You don't have room for everything, so you have to make priorities. I've got some new priorities now.

He realized that he could not manage everything and said that he would therefore prioritize his family in the future. Another participant put it more directly: "I want to be part of what's going on, be available, be there for the family".

Here there is little doubt that this prisoner expressed a clear desire to prioritize the family better.

For many of the participants, such prioritization involved taking responsibility: "You easily forget you're a father while you're inside, and this course gives you the energy to … you're a dad and you have to take responsibility".

This participant not only emphasized the importance of taking responsibility, he also pointed out how the fathering role is under-communicated in prisons, and that fatherhood was therefore a topic that inmates tend not to think about. Another participant said it this way:

> Well, it has been nice—but there's been too little about what you can do as a father in prison. Nevertheless, it has been a nice course. I have been looking forward to each meeting. It has been a nice group; everyone has been open—we have been able to talk about what's important for us.

This participant, like most others, emphasized the group processes within the participant group. This may also be an explanation of why the participants were very consistent in how they perceived the program.

Relationship to the family

The program did not only help the participants to change their priorities. It also led to a changed relationship with their family. When asked how his partner reacted to his joining the program, one prisoner replied: "She was very pleased, she can see I've taken a course. I've learned to communicate better with the kids and with her." Another informant provided a more detailed description of the new knowledge:

> I've really benefited from it, I hadn't seen my daughter for three years and I've been inside for two and a half years, and now I've been helped by the instructors, so they let me out on a temporary leave to meet her outside. I have worked at it a lot myself, but I've also been helped a lot. I call my daughter every week, and I've done that for two and a half years, but since I met her, it's gotten quite different. Before, I used to talk 80% of the time, but now she talks 80%. She's opened up and talks in a completely different way.

Some of the changes can of course be attributed to normal development in children, but there is little doubt that this participant gave the program credit for improved contact with his daughter. Others provided similar descriptions of how the program had either revived previous contact or established new contact, also with other family members than the participant's children. Another participant emphasized the importance of the program:

> The fun of this program is that I've thought that I'm in control of it ... I've been satisfied with my knowledge and then I started the course and then I understand that I've that what I thought is not nearby of how a father should have contact with his son.

New knowledge

The program has clearly also given the participants important knowledge of how to perform the role of a father.

> The course was very good. You learn about a lot of things you maybe know, but you quickly forget them. Like communication with kids. How to deal with children and so on. The kind of things people take for granted, but there's so much more. For example, it's important to make memories, to find things to do together. Going fishing for example. Bonding with the children. Doing things that aren't just fun for you.

This participant has clearly learned that in certain contexts the role of a father must be performed on the children's terms in order to create a good relationship. Another participant was more precise as to what he had learned:

I had only been married one year before I was put in, so I have received very much infor-mation I have needed—things like communication and problem solving. I have also learned a lot about children's development.

One participant provided the following reflection:

You get some thoughts in your head about going home. How I'm going to deal with situ-ations that crop up. I reckon I'll have to think through things … you do think a bit about how you want to appear to your kid. It should be kind of right for everyone. You need to find a balance to make it work.

The words of this participant were not as precise, but he was thinking along similar lines—it is important to create a balance between the needs and wishes of the children and the adults.

I've learned a lot about how to talk to the boy. He doesn't understand everything, but he's very keen to find out. He wonders a lot about what it's like here—how I'm getting on—if they're nice to me and things like that.

Communication is a key element of the program. For this father who had only had sporadic contact with his son in recent years, this knowledge was important. He also mentioned another point—the fear of children that their dad is suffering in prison.

Kids think of jail with bars and so on. He doesn't sleep well at night because he's thinking about me. That's the punishment that's taught me something. It would have been different if I'd been alone. But that's not possible now. So the family day was great. We had a meal together, we looked at the animals, and after four o'clock we could go off separately, each one to talk to his family alone.

The program includes a family day where the participants' families can visit them; here the participants themselves arrange different family activities. Of course, closed prisons place restrictions on the kind of activities that could be arranged, but this participant was in an open prison, which included a small farm. There is good reason to believe that the chil-dren's encounter with this prison reassured them that their father was fine despite being in prison. Another positive measure for the participants was the family quarters, or "visitors' house".

The visitors' house is a great deal, we get peace and quiet and I get time to talk to my wife too. I have a wife and three children. The visiting rooms here aren't suitable for that. I don't get time for each one of them—they can't all get the attention they deserve.

This participant also pointed out that visiting rooms in closed prisons are often poorly adapted to family visits. Another participant said it this way: "Visiting rooms should be made more family friendly. They are cramped … those who have kids need to get more visits." However, family days, where the family can see a much greater part of the prison, were experienced as positive in closed prisons.

As a consequence, the participants gained a different perspective on their lives: "I can see how much I'm missing, the kids are really number one. I don't want them to go through this again".

There were many who agreed with this conclusion; if they are to give their children proper attention, they have to choose a life without crime.

The problems of the family

If the father is in prison, it affects the whole family. The participants were fully aware of this.

> I can see how the situation has changed for my family—especially for the kids—they're struggling a bit—it would have been good if the course had focused a bit more on how to deal with the challenges the children face—what do you do if the children have problems at school, both social and learning problems.

> Our money's tight now. I worked a lot and earned good money and now she's sitting there and has to pay for the house, the cars, the caravan and so on. Now we have to count every cent. As we're not officially married, she doesn't get any support …

Several participants therefore pointed out the need to improve their domestic situation by finding solutions to poor finances, children's educational and social problems, and other challenges their family was facing. The father cannot solve these problems when he is in prison. Consequently, if the family is to receive help with these challenges, others must be involved. Some suggested that the mothers should be involved more in the program.

> [They could have] a talk on the phone with the family members, or a talk with the wives and girlfriends as a group. The instructors on the course get to know us and then they could have a talk together and get an idea of our home situation. There's no doubt that it's the ones outside who have the most problems and it would be good to have knowledge about that. How does this affect the kid and what can be done, not only by the prisoners, but also by the prison, to improve the situation for the children.

This statement points to an issue that concerned other participants: there are no procedures to address the problems faced by the family while the father is in prison. This is a challenge that the correctional services leave to others to relate to. Several of the participants felt that the program taught them too little about what they could do to help the family. Here are two examples:

> We need an overview of what rights we have and how to get these rights. It should have been automated that you got all the information that was relevant once you got into prison and they registered you were a father.

> The financial support for families with daddy in prison is bad, but there are some possibilities including extra child benefit after six months in prison—I had to figure it out my selves. The prison's social service did not know that.

Discussion

As described earlier, the main purpose of this program was to motivate participants to become more law-abiding. It has previously been shown that the program worked in line with that purpose (Hansen, 2017). Here it will be discussed whether the program also improved prisoners' fathering skills and limited the negative impact of the imprisonment on their families.

Strengthening the father's role

Feedback from the participants indicated that most of them, at least those with poor contact with their children, planned to participate more actively in family life. On the basis of studies conducted, we know that children with a father who is absent, both phys-ically and socially, may develop behavioral problems and poor mental health (Dowling & Gardner, 2005). If the program helps participants take greater responsibility and become actively involved in the well-being of their children and family, this will reduce the risk of negative developments in the children's situation. We naturally have no evidence that the fathers follow up on their ambitions after release; the choices made then will be influenced by a number of factors, only one of which will be the insight provided by the program. Nevertheless, we may assume that these fathers have a better basis for making the right choices after release as a result of this new insight.

Experience from many studies has shown that the social environment in prisons tends to be concerned with and emphasize quite different roles than that of a father (Christie, 2007; Grambo, 2000). This implies that being a father is not generally a topic discussed between inmates. The Norwegian Correctional Service has certainly implemented a number of measures in recent years to enhance contact between prisoners and their families, including visitors' houses in several prisons where inmates can stay with their family, often for 24 hours. There are also officers with responsibility for children to ensure that the visits are safe and in the best interests of the children. But in spite of this, prisoners still find it difficult to talk about their children and family with other inmates (Hansen et al., 2013). The "Fathers in Prison" program is therefore a setting where fatherhood is a legitimate topic of discussion, and can help participants become more aware of their responsibility towards their children both during and after their sentence.

The story of the prisoner who contacted his daughter after two and a half years in prison also shows that for some the program did actually lead to better contact with their children. There is therefore reason to believe that the program can reduce the risk of childhood behavioral problems due to lack of contact with the father (Dowling & Gardner, 2005; Murray et al., 2012). Lack of contact between fathers and children, both during and after the sentence, leads to various mental and social challenges for the chil-dren (Dallaire et al., 2010; Poehlmann et al., 2010; Shlafer & Poehlmann, 2010). We may assume that these challenges will be reduced when fathers establish regular contact with children with whom they have previously had occasional or no contact.

It is also important that participants report how they have acquired better parenting skills. This is especially true of those who do not have much experience with the role of the father. Partly, participants have gained knowledge of key issues such as child develop-ment, and partly they have been able to develop communication and problem solving skills. Several refer to partners having noted clear changes in the participants' behavior. The feedback also indicates that the open discussions in the group have helped to provide participants better insights into how to deal with the children the best way as possible.

A number of surveys of general parenting programs, outside the correctional services, show a clear correlation between increased parental competence and reduced risk behavior in children (see e.g. Sandler, Schoenfelder, Wolchik, & MacKinnon, 2011). Increased com-petence as a result of this program can therefore help fathers gain a broader perception of their fathering role. We know that many inmates have themselves had difficult childhoods (Friestad & Skog Hansen, 2004). They therefore do not necessarily have the same good role models to relate to as many other parents have had in their own parents. It thus seems probable that a program to improve fathering skills will be particularly effective for this target group.

Participatory activities, such as planning and implementing the family day, gave the participants experience in arranging activities with their children and family. There was clear feedback from the participants that they found it positive to gain experience of how activities with children must also take place on the children's own terms. The program thus enhanced the participants' competence in active participation in their children's upbringing, thus reducing the risks inherent in lack of involvement (Dowling & Gardner, 2005)

The decision by the father to change his way of life and desist from criminal activity is probably the most important factor in the long term. A number of studies conclude that improved contact between prisoner and family is the main contributing factor to a decision to turn away from criminal behavior (Hunter et al., 2013; Lösel et al., 2012). Our study participants also provided clear feedback that the focus on the family and insight into the harmful effect of their behavior on their children changed their attitude towards crime.

The conclusion is that the "Fathers in Prison" program helps fathers take greater responsibility for their children's situation, improves their interest in their children and enhances father–child contact. The program strengthens the fathers' ability to perform a fathering role both during and after imprisonment. However, it does not solve all the problems.

Lack of help for the family

Several prisoners called for better help in solving the problems that arise for their families. The participants reported that their families were unfamiliar with the existing support schemes and were insufficiently active in seeking help. One of the reasons why family members do not actively seek out relevant support may be the shame associated with having a family member in prison (Hardy & Snowden, 2010). Surveys of other groups have shown that it may be challenging to pinpoint the needs of users who are unclear about their needs themselves, and who also have negative experiences with public services. In such cases, it can be difficult to establish good relationships to enable those in need to formulate their needs and the kind of help they want (Hansen et al., 2013). It is difficult to imagine that the child of a prisoner who tries to hide the fact that his father is in prison would contact the school nurse to talk about his anxiety, social withdrawal and poor academic performance. For a number of children of prisoners, it is therefore crucial to ensure that there are support services that are aware of their challenges and have the time and desire to establish sufficient trust to enable children to open up about their problems. It does not seem possible to establish such services within the Norwegian Correctional Service. It is also clear that many of the families of inmates have a variety of different and complex problems. This therefore requires that the different agencies involved are not only individually aware of such challenges, but also see the need to engage in establishing comprehensive and coordinated services.

Prison fatherhood programs have been inspired by general parenting programs offered to parents outside prison. Some of these have also been provided to Norwegian prisoners with good results (Sherr, Skar, Clucas, von Tetzchner, & Hundeide, 2011). Internationally, one of the most successful parenting programs is the Triple P program. This uses a training program as a base, but offers more than training. In addition, during the training program, it is ascertained whether the participating families need other services, and if so, the instructors will contact relevant parties such as the school and health and social services. These will then jointly develop a plan for coordinated and comprehensive services for the family (Sanders, 2008).

A broad approach to the whole family's problems such as the Triple P program may therefore be a suitable strategy to be used in conjunction with "Fathers in Prison". It is therefore pertinent to consider a scheme which assesses the situation for both prisoner and family and involves collaboration with other players to address the problems of the entire family. However, only a small proportion of inmates participate in programs such as "Fathers in Prison". All the documentation available, both nationally and internationally, shows that families of prisoners are a high-risk group with a greater prevalence of financial problems, poor physical and mental health, learning difficulties and reduced social functioning (Farrington, 2005; Light & Campbell, 2007). Here there is a clearly defined group at risk calling for preventive measures.

We do not have a simple answer as to how to establish a comprehensive and coordinated intervention for prisoners' families, but the experience gained from this study strongly suggests that neither the correctional services nor the prisoners themselves can take sole responsibility to address this challenge. Such an intervention must largely be in the hands of non-prison services. It is therefore desirable that various other services pay particular attention to the challenges facing the families of prisoners. Public health nurses, teachers, child welfare, social services and general practitioners should focus on identifying the needs of this group and be prepared to collaborate with others to establish comprehensive and coordinated services (Hardy & Snowden, 2010).

The ambitions of the "Fathers in Prison" program to motivate and qualify the participants for an active fathering role have largely been fulfilled. This has had a positive effect on prisoners, their children and other family members, and has facilitated reintegration into the family and society as a whole (Lösel et al., 2012). The problems pointed out by the participants are thus not related to how fathers can be reintegrated after release. What the program does not solve are the key issues for the families while the father is in prison: financial problems, poor mental and physical health, stigmatization and social exclusion (Dolan, Loomes, Peasgood, & Tsuchiya, 2005; Hamsund & Sandvik, 2010).

If society wishes to reduce the burden on the families of prisoners, it must be understood that any measures taken by the correctional services or the prisoner will only have a limited effect. There must therefore be a stronger focus on what non-prison services can achieve. The key question is how relevant non-prison actors should work together to provide comprehensive and coordinated services to a proven high-risk group. Because prisoners' families have limited willingness and ability to request services themselves, it is necessary to be proactive towards them.

Disclosure statement

No potential conflict of interest was reported by the author.

References

Boswell, G. (2002). Imprisoned fathers: The children's view. *The Howard Journal of Criminal Justice, 41*(1), 14–26.

Christie, N. (2007). Sosial kontroll [Social control]. In L. Finstad, & C. Høigård (Eds.), *Kriminologi [Criminology]* (pp. 91–97). Oslo: Pax.

Christmann, K., Turliuc, M. N., & Mairean, C. (2012). Risk and resilience in children of prisoners: A research review. *Scientific Annals of the "Alexandru Ioan Cuza" University, Iaşi. New Series Sociology and Social Work Section, 5*(2), 115–137.

Dallaire, D. H., Ciccone, A., & Wilson, L. C. (2010). Teachers' experiences with and expectations of children with incarcerated parents. *Journal of Applied Developmental Psychology, 31*(4), 281–290.

Danermark, B., Ekström, M., Jacobsen, L., & Karlsson, J. C. (2003). *Att förklara samhället [Explaining society]*. Lund: Studentlitteratur.

Dolan, P., Loomes, G., Peasgood, T., & Tsuchiya, A. (2005). Estimating the intangible victim costs of violent crime. *The British Journal of Criminology, 45*, 958–976.

Dowling, S., & Gardner, F. (2005). Parenting programmes for improving the parenting skills and outcomes for incarcerated parents and their children. Protocol. The Cochrane Database of Systematic Reviews 2005. http://www.mrw.interscience.wiley.com/cochrane/clsysrev/articles/CD005557/frame.html

Egge, M. (2004). *De skjulte straffede [The hidden victims]*. Oslo: Redd Barna.

Farrington, D. P. (2005). Childhood origins of antisocial behavior. *Clinical Psychology & Psychotherapy, 12*(3), 177–190.

Ferraro, K., Johnson, J. M., Jorgensen, S., & Bolton, F. G. (1983). Problems of prisoners' families: The hidden costs of imprisonment. *Journal of Family Issues, 4*, 575–591.

Friestad, C., & Skog Hansen, I. L. (2004). *Levekår blant innsatte [Living conditions among inmates]*. Fafo Report 429. Oslo: Fafo.

Grambo, B. C. (2000). *Far og fange [Father and prisoner]*. (Dissertation). University of Oslo.

Hairston, C. F. (1989). Men in prison: Family characteristics and parenting views. *Journal of Offender Counseling Services and Rehabilitation, 14*, 23–30.

Hamsund, H., & Sandvik, A. B. (2010). De skjulte straffede – konsekvenser for pårørende når en i familien fengsles [The hidden victims: Consequences for the family when one member is imprisoned]. In L. Nilsen et al. (Eds.), *Det sårbare mennesket [The vulnerable human being]* (pp. 117–129). Stavanger: Hertervig.

Hansen, G. V. (2017). "Fathers in prison" program may create a basis for desistance among Norwegian prisoners. *Journal of Offender Rehabilitation, 56*(3), 173–187. doi:10.1080/10509674.2017.1290008

Hansen, G. V., Arvesen, P. A., & Tonholm, T. (2013): *Evaluering av programmet "Pappa i fengsel" [An evaluation of the "Fathers in Prison" program]*. Commissioned report. Halden: Østfold University College.

Hansen, G. V., & Samuelsen, F. (2016). Assessment of offenders: New trends in Norway. *EuroVista, 4*(2), 12–24.

Hardy, T., & Snowden, M. (2010). Familial impact of imprisonment and the community specialist practitioner. *Community Practitioner, 83*(10), 21–25.

Hoffmann, H. C., Byrd, A. L., & Kightlinger, A. M. (2010). Prison programs and services for incarcerated parents and their underage children: Results from a national survey of correctional facilities. *The Prison Journal, 90*(4), 397–416.

Hunter, G., Skrine, O., Turnbull, P., Kazimirski, A., & Pritchard, D. (2013). *Intermediate outcomes of family and intimate relationship interventions: A rapid evidence assessment*. London: Institute for Criminal Policy Research and New Philanthropy Capital, National Offender Management Service.

Jones, A., Gallagher, B., Manby, M., Robertson, O., Schützwohl, M., Berman, A. H., & Christmann, K. (2013). *Children of prisoners: Interventions and mitigations to strengthen mental health*. Huddersfield: University of Huddersfield Repository.

Kvale, S. (2001). *Det kvalitative forskningsintervju [The qualitative research interview]*. Oslo: Gyldendal Akademisk.

Light, R., & Campbell, B. (2007). Prisoners' families: Still forgotten victims? *Journal of Social Welfare and Family Law, 28*(3–4), 297–308.

Loper, A. B., & Tuerk, E. H. (2006). Parenting programs for incarcerated parents: Current research and future directions. *Criminal Justice Policy Review, 17*(4), 407–427.

Lösel, F., Pugh, G., Markson, L., Souza, K., & Lanskey, C. (2012). *Risk and protective factors in the resettlement of imprisoned fathers with their families*. Ipswich: Ormiston Children's and Families Trust.

Malterud, K. (2012). Systematic text condensation: A strategy for qualitative analysis. *Scandinavian Journal of Public Health, 40*(8), 795–805.

Matthews, J. (1983). *Forgotten victims*. London: NACRO.

Morris, P. (1965). *Prisoners and their families*. London: Allen & Unwin.

Murray, J., Farrington, D. P., & Sekol, I. (2012). Children's antisocial behavior, mental health, drug use, and educational performance after parental incarceration: A systematic review and meta-analysis. *Psychological Bulletin, 138*(2), 175–210.

Poehlmann, J., Dallaire, D., Loper, A. B., & Shear, L. D. (2010). Children's contact with their incarcerated parents: Research findings and recommendations. *American Psychologist, 65*(6), 575–598.

Prochaska, J. O., & DiClemente, C. C. (1982). Transtheoretical therapy: Toward a more integrative model of change. *Psychotherapy: Theory, Research & Practice, 19*(3), 276–288.

Purvis, M. (2013). Paternal incarceration and parenting programs in prison: A review paper. *Psychiatry, Psychology and Law, 20*(1), 9–28.

Rollnick, S., & Miller, W. R. (1995). What is motivational interviewing? *Behavioural and Cognitive Psychotherapy, 23*(04), 325–334.

Ronel, N., & Segev, D. (2014). Positive criminology in practice. *International Journal of Offender Therapy and Comparative Criminology, 58*(11), 1389–1407.

Sanders, M. R. (2008). Triple P-Positive Parenting Program as a public health approach to strengthening parenting. *Journal of Family Psychology, 22*(4), 506–517.

Sandler, I. N., Schoenfelder, E. N., Wolchik, S. A., & MacKinnon, D. P. (2011). Long-term impact of prevention programs to promote effective parenting: Lasting effects but uncertain processes. *Annual Review of Psychology, 62*, 299–329.

Sherr, L., Skar, A.-M. S., Clucas, C., von Tetzchner, S., & Hundeide, K. (2011). *Evaluering av Program for foreldreveiledning basert på International Child Development Programme, Norsk sammendrag [Evaluation of parental guidance Programs based on the International Child Development Programme. Summary in Norwegian]*, Report to the Ministry of Children, Equality and Social Inclusion. Oslo: Ministry of Children, Equality and Social Inclusion.

Shlafer, R. J., & Poehlmann, J. (2010). Attachment and caregiving relationships in families affected by parental incarceration. *Attachment & Human Development, 12*(4), 395–415.

Smith, R., Grimshaw, R., Romeo, R., & Knapp, M. (2007). *Poverty and disadvantage among prisoners' families* (Vol. 10). York: Joseph Rowntree Foundation.

Stortingsmelding/Parlamentary White Paper No. 37. (2007–2008). *Straff som virker – mindre kriminalitet – tryggere samfunn [Punishment that works – Less crime – A safer society]*. Oslo: Ministry of Justice and Public Security.

Imprisoned Fathers and their Children: A Reflection on Two Decades of Research

Gwyneth Boswell*

ABSTRACT
Twenty years ago, the author co-led an extensive study for the UK Department of Health on the parenting role of imprisoned fathers in England and Wales. Against a background of children's needs and rights, it examined the place of fatherhood in their lives, the meaning of paternal absence to a child, and the particular significance for children of a father who was absent by reason of imprisonment. The study also looked at the effect of a father's imprisonment on the children's mothers/other carers, and upon the fathers themselves. It chronicled the range of facilities available to children to help them maintain contact with their father during his imprisonment. Not unlike earlier pioneers in this research field it concluded that, despite pockets of good practice depending largely on the interest of individual prison staff and the voluntary sector, this group of children remained under-prioritised and ill-supported by statutory child care and criminal justice policy and practice. Over the last two decades, research has continued on the topic of imprisoned fathers and their children but it seems that, with honourable exceptions, little has changed for them during this period. This brief reflection addresses the possible reasons for this deficit in England and Wales, the lack of official statistical information, the shortage of longitudinal research, and the politicisation of crime. Recommendations surrounding research and planning, and the enhancement of public understanding, are proposed.

Introduction

Between the years 1996 and 1998, the author co-led an extensive study in England and Wales, entitled "The Parenting Role of Imprisoned Fathers" (Boswell & Wedge, 1999, 2002) under the Department of Health's Research Initiative on "Supporting Parents" (Quinton, 2004). It conducted interviews with 181 men from geographically spread prison establishments (including six Young Offender Institutions) with 127 partners/child carers, 17 children of varied ages, and 16 prison staff running fathering courses and visiting provisions. Within an overall context of children's needs and rights, it

---

*Author's note: I am grateful to an anonymous reviewer for contemporary information about policy and practice in the U.S.A.

examined the meaning for them of a father, whether present or absent, and studied in particular the significance for those whose father was absent because of imprisonment.

The same study examined the effect of a father's imprisonment on the children's mothers/other carers, and upon the fathers themselves. It set out the range of facilities available to help children maintain contact with their father during his imprisonment. It concluded that, notwithstanding pockets of good practice depending largely on the interest of individual prison staff and the voluntary sector, this group of children remained under-prioritised and ill-supported by statutory child care and criminal justice policy and practice.

Earlier pioneers in this field, notably Morris (1965), Shaw (1987, 1992) and Richards (1992) had identified very similar factors in their research, highlighting the significant disadvantages for and additional practical and emotional needs of prisoners' children. Shaw, in particular, posed ethical and human rights questions:

> Does the state have a right morally—as practice shows it has legally—to strip a child of its parent because that parent has offended, although the crime may have been less harmful to the victim than the imprisonment of the offender is to his or her child? Does not the child have a right to uninterrupted parenting at least equal to the right of the state to punish? (Shaw, 1992, p. 195)

In their Scottish study, Peart and Asquith had concluded that "for most children imprisonment of a parent is a traumatic experience … .Feelings of loss and confusion may well be compounded by the altered financial and emotional resources of the remaining parent or carer". As a result, "the emphasis should shift from re-establishing family contact to maintaining family contact" (Peart & Asquith, 1992, pp. 21–22).

The opening up of UK-based research on imprisoned fathers and their children, as well as on imprisoned mothers (Catan, 1989; Lloyd, 1992) coincided to an extent with prison disturbances reported upon by Lord Justice Woolf and Judge Tumim (Home Office, 1991). The report made a number of recommendations in respect of family ties: increased home leave opportunities; sentences served in prisons closer to home; increased prison visits; and the consideration of extended prison visits with fathers and children. The Government of the time responded with a series of measures to implement the Woolf/Tumim recommendations, albeit that some constituted existing Home Office policy which, in practice, had been ignored (Shaw & Crook, 1991)

It was in this climate of renewed interest in relationships between prisoners and their families that other U.K.-based research and, in parallel, American and other European studies began to develop a wider published profile. In the U.S.A., Hairston's review of existing evidence, including that from the U.K., confirmed that many imprisoned fathers had played some kind of care-giving/nurturing role in their children's lives before incarceration, and they and their children wished this to continue. In line with U.K. developments of the time (e.g. NEPACS, 1997), research in the U.S.A. often brought together academics, professionals and lay people in a campaigning approach to support these relationships. Thus, a special issue of *Child Welfare: Journal of Policy, Practice and Program*, emanating from an initiative by the Child Welfare League of America, devoted itself to the subject of "Children with Parents in Prison" (Seymour & Hairston, 1998). In Europe, in 1993, the "European Action Research Committee on Children of Imprisoned Parents" (now "Children of Prisoners Europe"), funded by the Bernard

Van Leer Foundation, was set up, aiming both to represent the children's voice, and to explore child-centred approaches to maintaining the child–parent bond within European countries (Ayre, Philbrick, & Reiss, 2006).

However, while the renewed interest by researchers, professionals and voluntary organisations crossed from the last decade of the twentieth century into the first decade of the twenty-first century, it had not succeeded in transferring its findings and accompanying concerns and recommendations to Government policy in England and Wales. As our own studies of prisoner-fathers and their children continued during this period, we found that, following Woolf/Tumim, while some facilities were improved, others were worse than before, and others still awaiting improvement. Depressingly, we found ourselves at research conferences listening to accounts of contemporary (usually small-scale) research findings, which showed overall that little had changed for children and families since we reported at the turn of the century.

As a researcher, observer and commentator during and beyond the period chronicled above, I surmise that there are three main reasons for the apparent inability of research findings, professional, voluntary, and campaigning activity to convert to Government policy. These are: the lack of relevant statistical information; the shortage of longitudinal research to identify reliable outcomes for the maintenance of prisoner-father and child relationships; and the politicisation of crime from the 1990s onwards, with its accompanying need for more strategic and effective researcher-politician and researcher-public engagement. The subsequent sections will address each of these elements in turn.

The lack of relevant statistical information

The prison population in England and Wales has been rising steadily since 1940, when it stood at 9,377 (Allen & Watson, 2017). In March 2001, the prison population in England and Wales reached 65,394, of which 94.6% were men and 5.4% were women (Home Office, 2001). Although crime rates have declined over this period, the numbers imprisoned have steadily increased, reaching a record high in December 2011 of 88,179 (95.4% men; 4.6% women) following the August 2010 riots (Berman, 2012). By May 2017, the numbers imprisoned had fallen somewhat to 85,193—still 95.4% men and 4.6% women (Prison Population Statistics, 2017). It nevertheless remains the case that England and Wales has the highest rate of imprisonment in Western Europe per 100,000 of the population (Council of Europe, 2017) though, as Allen and Watson (2017) point out, international comparisons should be viewed with some caution due to differential criminal justice and counting systems.

As the foregoing paragraph demonstrates, there exist a good number of categories of information about prison populations. However, when it comes to information about the children of these populations which, in the case of England and Wales and some others, have been increasing exponentially, no official record exists. Neither prison reception staff, nor other involved criminal justice or social services ask routinely for this information. Yet, for as long as this author can remember, researchers, practitioners and campaigning groups, have been asking relevant ministries to make provision for the collection of data, firstly about the numbers of prisoners with children, and secondly the numbers of these children. Very few countries do this, Sweden being a notable exception within Europe, and some level of information being available in the United States where it was reported in 2007 that 52% of state inmates and 63% of federal inmates had children (Glaze & Maruschak, 2008) and in 2010, with a heavily rising prison population, that 2.7 million children had a parent behind bars (Western and Pettit, 2010). In England and Wales, the National Offender Management Service (N.O.M.S.) established in 2004 under New Labour, almost reached the point of incorporating this information category into its proposed new computerised database, but when that system failed, the impetus was lost. It remains to be seen whether the Conservative Government's successor to N.O.M.S., Her Majesty's Prison and Probation Service, launched in April 2017, will deem such information sufficiently important to seek to incorporate it into its data-collecting processes in the future.

In the meantime, those who seek to research and practice in the field of prisoners and families are obliged to rely on estimated numbers of children experiencing parental imprisonment. Over time, and as prison populations in England and Wales have grown, these have included 100,000 (Shaw, 1987); 125,000 (Ramsden, 1998); 125,000–150,000 (Murray & Farrington, 2008); and 200,000 (Ministry of Justice, 2010). Barnardo's (2014) suggests that in relation to imprisoned parents in Northern Ireland's three prisons, "1,500 children are affected on any given day"; and in relation to Scotland's 15 prisons, "30,000 children face parental imprisonment every year". As these figures make apparent, there is at present no consistent mechanism for arriving at these kinds of estimates. Further, apart from Shaw's, (1987) estimate, which was based on a survey of 415 men in one English prison, no other U.K.-based estimates have differentiated between children of mothers and children of fathers. Indeed there are many problems associated with the extrapolation of such information, including the fact that women in particular may not disclose that they have children, for fear of them being taken into care, though systematic cross-agency communication such as between prisons and kinship support services could mitigate this drawback (Boswell & Wood, 2011). Crucially, therefore, and with a small number of exceptions (for example, Boswell, 2002; Brown, 2001) the voice of the child, because of lack of identification, is rarely heard.

The negative effects of parental imprisonment upon children are, by now, well-chronicled, and it is not the purpose of this article to recount them. However, it is worth referring here to the meaning of fatherhood for children, in order to highlight its importance for the estimated numbers of children with imprisoned fathers whose lack of, or reduction in paternal contact may be impacting on their psycho-social development. The social construction of fatherhood has gradually changed since the end of World War Two. From being barely-mentioned in pre-1970s childcare literature, other than as providers and disciplinarians, fathers' involvement in child-rearing has slowly come to be acknowledged. This has become manifest for example, in their involvement in childbirth, their role in children's play and sport, and their increased sharing of childcare within the family since the majority of mothers now go out to work. A contemporary survey by the Modern Family Index reported that 69% of fathers said they would consider their childcare arrangements before they took a new job or promotion (Bright Horizons and Working Families, 2017). From the 1990s onwards, researchers were moving beyond the concept of role, to look at the actual nature of father–child interaction. In a review of fathers and fatherhood in Britain, Burghes, Clarke, and Cronin (1997) chose to ask the question "What do fathers and children do together?", while Milligan and Dowie (1998) asked "What do Children Need from their Fathers?". Their research, based in

Scotland, drew on cross-class groups of 58 fathers and mothers and 67 children, concluding that the reality was one of underlying subtlety:

> Without prejudice to the view that mothers can provide their children with more or less anything that fathers might give, at a more fundamental level, there is still one need which it seems **only** a father can meet, and this is not a truism—namely **the apparent need of** daughters and sons to have a satisfactory and unproblematic relationship specifically with that one person who is uniquely their father (Milligan & Dowie, 1998, p. 65).

The need for that unique relationship, assuming that it has not been assessed as damaging to the child, is no different for children of imprisoned fathers than for any other children. Strained though that need is for children of any absent father, it is even more so for those with fathers in prison, who have the physical and psychological walls of a forbidding institution to contend with. Researchers in the U.S.A. examined the relationship between paternal incarceration and developmental outcomes for approximately 3000 urban children. They concluded:

> The estimated effects of paternal incarceration on the psychological, social and economic development of children are stronger than those of other forms of father absence, suggesting that children with incarcerated fathers may require specialized support from caretakers, teachers, and social service providers (Geller, Cooper, Garfinkel, Schwartz-Soicher, & Mincy, 2012).

As Barnardo's report on identifying and supporting children with a parent in prison observes, however:

> Without a sensitive understanding of the numbers of children involved, it is impossible to assess the extent of services that they need to address the issues they face and deliver the prompt support that we know makes a difference to each child (Barnardo's, 2014, p. 8).

Barnardo's calls for the Ministry of Justice to appoint a lead minister to have responsibility for children of prisoners. They suggest that such a minister would be responsible for both the identification of such children and for the development of a National Action Plan to support such children via a multi-agency approach. They would be identified by the placing of a statutory duty upon courts to establish whether those committed to prison have children and, if so, whether any immediate care arrangements which have been put in place are satisfactory. A review of the Scottish Government's commitments in the same field carried the follow-up recommendation that that Government "should carry out Children's Rights Impact Assessments on all initiatives, policies and guidance publications that affect the rights of children of offenders" (SCCYP, 2011, p. 13)

Finally, in the light of ever-increasing prison populations across Europe and the U.S.A., it is clear that, as Murray and Farrington (2008) suggest, large-scale surveys are needed in order to accurately assess the current and cumulative prevalence of children experiencing parental imprisonment. Further, since most prison populations comprise an overwhelming majority of men, and disproportionate numbers of black and ethnic minority prisoners (see, for example, The Lammy Review, 2017; The White House, 2015), such studies need clearly to distinguish between male and female prisoner-parents, and between ethnic groups, in order to determine the differential needs of their children. These suggested developments would enable researchers to deliver clearer and more reliable messages to governments as to the type and extent of measures required to safeguard the well-being of children with fathers in prison.

The shortage of longitudinal research

Over the last 30 years, a great deal of qualitative research has been conducted in many countries on the circumstances of prisoners' children and families. These studies provide important accounts of the ways in which children may experience parental imprisonment and how it may affect them. None, to the author's knowledge, has concluded anything other than that the majority of children, along with their families, are economically, physically and emotionally disadvantaged, and receive little support from statutory agencies, though many examples of good individual and voluntary agency-based practice are reported. In some cases, visiting arrangements have improved physically but, in terms of what really counts to families—the atmosphere and the levels of respect with which they are, or are not, treated by staff—the visiting environment remains very variable.

Parenting programmes and family and kinship support projects have been more of a success story in terms of their reported positive impact on both young and adult prisoners, partners and children (for example, Boswell, Poland, & Moseley, 2011; Boswell & Poland, 2009; Boswell, Wedge, & Price, 2005; Dominey, Dodds, & Wright, 2016). Some of these studies provide short-term outcome data in terms of attitude, behaviour, parenting styles and early impact on children. For practical reasons, however, most are unable to identify a comparison group of the general population (Murray, Farrington, Sekol, & Olsen, 2009).

Other U.K.-based research, which has looked more widely at outcomes over periods of up to one year, include a study of prisoners' childhoods and family backgrounds with a cohort of 3849 prisoners (Ministry of Justice, 2014); and a study of risk and protective factors in 358 data cases associated with the resettlement of imprisoned fathers and their families (Lösel, Pugh, Markson, Souza, & Lanskey, 2012). It is rare, however, for funding to be made available for researchers to embark upon long-term prospective longitudinal studies. A small number of retrospective studies have managed to draw upon more general longitudinal data to identify specific outcomes for children of imprisoned parents (not distinguished by gender) as against outcomes for control groups without this parental experience. In the U.S.A., for example, Kjellstrand and Eddy (2011) utilised existing data on adolescent youth to examine the family context and later problematic behaviour in young people who had experienced the incarceration of a parent in childhood. In the U.K., Murray drew on Farrington's well-known longitudinal Cambridge study of 411 boys, to identify outcomes for 23 boys who had experienced parental imprisonment as against four control groups of those who had not (Murray & Farrington, 2005). In both cases, and in keeping with most other studies on the topic, parental imprisonment during childhood proved to be a strong predictor of adverse, including delinquent and anti-social outcomes through the life course.

The importance of longitudinal studies is their ability to document change from one point in time to another, and to yield more reliable and valid data than can single-point studies. They also have the advantage of being able to engender trust over time between researchers and a sometimes wary, often stigmatised, respondent group increasing the potential for eliciting reliable data. Thus, Farrington has been able to follow up his cohort at key points for nearly 60 years and importantly to identify both risk and protective factors for future delinquency. A 12-year longitudinal study, annually following up male teenage sex offenders who had been resident in a therapeutic community, documented both their low re-offending rates against a comparison group, and also how, over time, they had developed stable lifestyles, often based on learning from their therapeutic experience (Boswell, Wedge, Moseley, Dominey, & Poland, 2016). As a consequence of change being assessed both quantitatively and qualitatively over time, it is possible more accurately to pinpoint potential causes of particular behaviours and thus to identify for policy and practice, the measures that are most appropriate for preventing negative outcomes.

However, the general lack of availability of funds to study the field for much longer than a year is probably a reflection of negligible levels of public and ministerial interest in the plight of prisoners' children as compared, for example, with the extent of research material on children of separation and divorce. In the case of prisoner fathers, this may also relate to the "deficit" model of fatherhood often applied to those who may be assumed, without evidence, to be "bad fathers" (Hawkins & Dollahite, 1997). Thus, it is difficult to gauge levels of impact of this experience for children over a meaningful period, say three to five years after a prisoner's release. Yet almost everything that has been chronicled over the last 30 years of research activity suggests that the effects of imprisonment upon children require this length of large-scale examination, both to identify and mitigate negative outcomes over time, and importantly also to point to appropriate support systems to a vulnerable and often overlooked population.

The politicisation of crime

The foregoing sections have hinted at the difficulty of obtaining political attention for the children of prisoners. As Winston Churchill famously said, while Home Secretary: "The mood and temper of the public in regard to the treatment of crime and criminals is one of the most unfailing tests of the civilisation of any country." In the same speech he went on to express a belief in rehabilitation and "an unfaltering faith that there is a treasure, if only you can find it in the heart of every person" (Hansard, 1910). Prior to the early 1990s, a broadly liberal political outlook by all parties on penal policy, which had tended to keep all but the most heinous crimes out of the public eye, had continued to obtain. Indeed in a White Paper at the start of that decade, the Conservative Home Secretary, Douglas Hurd described prison as "an expensive way of making bad people worse" (Home Office, 1990).

In 1992, however, there was a public outcry at the murder of two-year-old James Bulger by two ten-year-old boys, and during their subsequent high-profile trial. Little was done to promote public understanding of the possible reasons for their behaviour; sensationalism ruled in the shape of photographs and captions portraying these two children as "born evil". Although other children had committed murder, few had reached the headlines in this dramatic way, and its coverage did much to generate a more punitive attitude towards crime and criminals generally. This culminated in a highly-publicised speech by the Home Secretary, Michael Howard, to the Conservative Party Conference in 1993, claiming that "prison works". Since then, as noted earlier, the impact on prison populations has been dramatic, the numbers almost doubling over the subsequent two and a half decades. During this period, crime has been increasingly politicised worldwide, and its perpetrators and all those associated with them have become even more unpopular than hitherto. This, of course, relates partly to the wide-reaching aftermath of events such as the al Qaida attacks on the U.S. World Trade Center on 11 September

2001 and their subsequent smaller-scale replication in other capital cities, followed by the rise of radicalisation and terrorism on the part of a range of insurgent groups, notably I.S.I.L. As a consequence, the preservation of security at every level has become paramount, including within prisons, in many of which children and prisoner-parents are no longer allowed physical contact, despite the best efforts of voluntary and campaigning organisations such as Action for Prisoners' Families, the Ormiston Trust, the Prison Reform Trust and the Howard League. Other momentous world events such as the Rwandan genocide in 1994 also had its consequences for prisoners' children. In a visit to Rwandan prisons overflowing with "genocidaires" in 2002, our research team discovered that children and families were allowed to visit only for 3 minutes and had to stand on one side of a line while the prisoners stood on the other, with no touching allowed.

During the course of our own national study, 18 years of a Conservative Government with a hard-line Home Secretary at its helm for its last few years, was replaced by a New Labour administration also determined to be "tough on crime", though never, seemingly "tough on the causes of crime" its accompanying epithet, which might have led to some change for prisoners' families. Instead, the punitive political climate of the preceding era was left to continue in the shape of the gradual demise of the statutory criminal justice services, notably the probation service, and in the growing struggle for the voluntary sector to obtain funding to run services for prisoners and families:

> Although families are recognised as playing a role within the rehabilitative process, in a climate of retribution families become part of the landscape of punishment of the offender for wrongdoing. Limitations on contact with one's family becomes part of the retributive experience. The "permeable wall" between prison and the outside community envisaged in Woolf's vision of community prisons has failed to materialise .... By implication, the response of criminal justice agencies to the needs of prisoners' families indicates symbolic denunciation not only of the offender, but also of his or her family (Codd, 1998, p. 152).

On assuming power in May 2010, the Conservative-led Coalition Government's priority was to make deep spending cuts across most ministries, including the Ministry of Justice, set up by the previous administration. Despite his initial enthusiasm for a (cost-saving) "Rehabilitation Revolution" set out in a Green Paper (Ministry of Justice, 2010), the first Coalition Justice Minister, Kenneth Clarke, was obliged by his harder-line colleagues to quash proposals to reduce the number of people sentenced to prison over the next 3 years. His successors in a Conservative administration since 2015 have done little to further the cause of rehabilitation. Such public monies as were once available to spend on visitors' centres, crèches, the staffing of extended visits, parenting programmes, family and kinship support work and the like, became severely curtailed and liable to be subject to a newly-introduced "Payment by Results" policy. In the case of children and families, the most important outcome measure appeared likely to be whether or not the prisoner is re-convicted, rather than or at least equal to the maintained/improved well-being of the child. In terms of the rights of the child, this is probably the lowest point reached by criminal justice policy since our own researches began some 20 years ago.

Research-informed action for children and prisoner-fathers

To increase the chances of the implementation of research findings about the adverse effect upon children with imprisoned fathers, and the benefits of a range of services for them, it is necessary for researchers to engage more effectively with both politicians and the general public (Sedgeman, 2017). This is likely to require a considerable dose of pragmatism. Ministers, who make and influence policy, have extremely busy lives, and tend to be lobbied from all sides. It is worth researching whether they are the best people to approach, or whether action is more likely to follow from submission of evidence to a Select Committee or to an influential member of the House of Lords, for example. Committee rooms in both Houses can be hired for presentations and relevant Members invited. In whichever form evidence is presented, and to whomever, it is important always to make available a single-sided sheet of paper preferably in large font, starting with a single-eye-catching message, followed by no more than two or three main findings, with clear (and preferably costed) suggestions for how they could be delivered in practice. Politicians are always conscious of their poll ratings, so to get clear policy ideas out into the public arena, persuasive communication is needed. Based on the reflections within this paper, the following suggestions are tendered.

Research and planning

Policy-makers in this arena have to balance society's need for justice, retribution and protection with children's needs and rights to sustain contact and, thereby, loving and meaningful relationships with their incarcerated parent. In the interests both of the children's future emotional stability and of discovering more about the links between sustained family ties and subsequent reoffending, it is apparent that further longitudinal research needs to be funded and conducted. It would be valuable to know, for example, how effectively prisoners returning to their families are able to assume the role of responsible parent at home—to the best advantage of their children. This type of information should be fully integrated into policy formation with a mutual exchange which entails policy-makers facilitating the collection of important demographic information for researchers in the field. In the U.S.A., the 2002–8 Obama administration instigated an unprecedented research-based focus on children of the incarcerated, leading to major funding and policy initiatives in the Departments of Justice and Health and Human Services, moving to policy and programme development at State level. This kind of development highlights the necessity to make research frameworks international, so that action can be informed by successes and failures elsewhere, to save scarce resources and avoid "reinventing the wheel".

The enhancement of public understanding

The general public is justifiably concerned about, and sometimes fearful of, prisoners, prisons and all of those associated with them. They need to understand that to ascribe negative labels to prisoners' families, and their children in particular, is not to solve the problem but to perpetuate it; they, too, are entitled to hear serious rather than salacious facts which may help them form more objective and ultimately more compassionate and supportive attitudes. Public relations have never been the strong suit of the criminal justice system; the politicisation of crime has, to some extent, obviated the need for it. Researchers, practitioners and campaigners can all work more strategically to inform politicians and the public both about the needs and rights of prisoners' children, in the way that, for example, the "See Us, Support Us" campaign is doing in the U.S.A. (The Osborne Association, 2015), while crucially stressing the importance for long-term community safety of supporting released prisoners' reintegration into their families and communities.

Statutory compulsion

As is well-known, measures to support the human rights of children to maintain contact with a parent from whom they are separated are enshrined in the U.N. Convention on the Rights of the Child, 1989; the principle of respect for family life is incorporated in the European Convention on Human Rights. Most countries, with the notable exception of the U.S.A., have ratified the former and included the latter in human rights legislation, but many, including the U.K., have been slow, and probably reluctant, to apply these measures to prisoners' children. Nevertheless, case law and Children's Ombudsmen have the power to challenge this, and campaigning organisations such as The Howard League (2017) have shown that rights-based legal challenges against, for example, legal aid cuts affecting children, and the solitary confinement of children in custody can be won. Advocacy measures, such as those supported by the Bill of Rights for Children of Incarcerated Parents employed at State level in the U.S.A. (San Francisco, 2005) and The Regional Platform for the Defense of the Rights of Children of Incarcerated Parents in Latin American and the Caribbean (NNAPES, 2015) have been successfully brought to bear by lawyers on matters relating to parental imprisonment in those countries. The Scottish Sentencing Council (2017) has very recently discussed adopting a "best interests of the child" approach (though arguably this is subtly different to a children's rights basis) to the sentencing of parents. All of these measures demonstrate the potential for children's rights properly to be taken into account in England and Wales, across the wider U.K. and beyond, whether in the employment of the law, or in developing codes of practice at all stages of the justice process where parental imprisonment is under consideration.

Conclusion

This article has reflected on the ways in which policy and provision for children and their imprisoned fathers in England and Wales have and have not changed over the last 20 years. Despite cumulative bodies of research findings to the effect that prisoners' children and families suffer considerable hardship, but that they can benefit from a range of programmes set up to support them and their family ties, Governments, the media and, thereby, public opinion remain unconvinced. It will take effective, pragmatic communication from researchers to politicians and the public, based on reliable statistics, hard evidence, and ideally statutory compulsion to bring about lasting change to this neglected section of society.

Disclosure statement

No potential conflict of interest was reported by the author.

References

Allen, G., & Watson, C. (2017). *UK prison population statistics: Briefing paper number SN/SG/ 04334, 20 April 2017*. London: House of Commons Library.

Ayre, L., Philbrick, K., & Reiss, M. (Eds.). (2006). *Children of imprisoned parents: European perspectives on good practice*. Paris: Eurochips.

Barnardo's. (2014). *On the outside: Identifying and supporting children with a parent in prison*. Ilford: Auhor.

Berman, G. (2012). *Prison population statistics: Standard note SN/SG/4334*. Social and General Statistics. London: House of Commons Library.

Boswell, G. (2002). Imprisoned Fathers: The children's view. *The Howard Journal of Criminal Justice, 41*(1), 14–26.

Boswell, G., & Poland, F. (2009). *Review of the levels of implementation and learning progression by graduates of two prison parenting and family relationship programmes*. London: Safe Ground.

Boswell, G., Poland, F., & Moseley, A. (2011). *The 'family man' impact study: An evaluation of the longer-term effectiveness of safe ground's revised family relationships programme on prisoner graduates, their supporters and families*. London: Safe Ground.

Boswell, G., & Wedge, P. (1999). *The parenting role of imprisoned fathers*. London: Official Report to the Dept. of Health.

Boswell, G., & Wedge, P. (2002). *Imprisoned fathers and their children*. London & Philadelphia: Jessica Kingsley Publishers.

Boswell, G., Wedge, P., & Price, A. (2005). The impact of fathers inside. Evaluation of an OLSU/safe ground parenting course for adult male prisoners. *Prison Service Journal*, May; *159*, 7–11.

Boswell, G., & Wood, M. (2011). *An evaluation of the effectiveness of pact's kinship care support service at HMP Holloway*. London: Prison Advice and Care Trust.

Boswell, G. R., Wedge, P., Moseley, A., Dominey, J., & Poland, F. (2016). Treating sexually harmful teenage males: A summary of longitudinal research findings on the effectiveness of a therapeutic community. *The Howard Journal of Crime and Justice, 55*(1-2), 168–187.

Bright Horizons and Working Families. (2017). *The modern family index, 2017*. London: Author.

Brown, K. (2001). *"No-one's ever asked me": Young people with a prisoner in the family*. London: Federation of Prisoners' Families' Support Groups.

Burghes, L., Clarke, L., & Cronin, N. (1997). *Fathers and fatherhood in Britain*. London: Family Policy Studies Institute.

Catan, L. (1989). The development of young children in HMP mother and baby units. *Home Office Research Bulletin, 26*, 9–12.

Codd, H. (1998). 'Prisoners' families: The "forgotten victims". *Probation Journal, 45*(3), 148–154.

Council of Europe. (2017). *Annual penal statistics. Survey 2015, Updated on 25th April 2017*. Strasbourg: Space 1 – Prison Populations: Council of Europe.

Dominey, J., Dodds, C., & Wright, S. (2016). *Bridging the Gap: A review of the pact family engagement service*. London: Prison Advice and Care Trust.

Geller, A., Cooper, C. E., Garfinkel, I., Schwartz-Soicher, O., & Mincy, R. B. (2012). Beyond absenteeism: Father incarceration and child development. *Demography, 49*(1), 49–76.

Glaze, L., & Maruschak, L. (2008). *Parents in prison and their minor children*. Washington, DC: Bureau of Justice Statistics (Special Report).

Hansard. (1910). *HC deb 20 July 1910 vol 19 cc1354*. London: Hansard, House of Commons.

Hawkins, A., & Dollahite, D. (1997). *Generative fathering: Beyond deficit perspectives*. London: Sage.

Home Office. (1990). *Crime justice and protecting the public*. Cm 965. London: HMSO.

Home Office. (1991). *Report into prison disturbances April 1990 by the right honourable justice Woolf and his honour, Judge Stephen Tumim*. Cm 1456. London: HMSO.

Home Office. (2001). *Occupation of prisons and remand centres, young offender institutions and police cells, England and Wales, 31 March 2001.* London: Research, Development and Statistics Directorate – Offenders and Corrections Unit.

Kjellstrand, J., & Eddy, J. (2011). Parental incarceration during childhood, family context, and youth problem behavior across adolescence. *Journal of Offender Rehabilitation,* Jan 1; 50(1), 18–36.

Lloyd, E. (Ed.). (1992). *Children visiting Holloway prison: Inside and out perspectives on the all-day visits scheme at HMP Holloway.* London: Save the Children.

Lösel, F., Pugh, G., Markson, L., Souza, K., & Lanskey, C. (2012). *Risk and protective factors in the resettlement of imprisoned fathers with their families.* Milton: Ormiston Children's and Families Trust.

Milligan, C., & Dowie, A. (1998). *What do children need from their fathers?* Occasional paper no. 42: University of Edinburgh: Centre for Theology and Public Issues.

Ministry of Justice. (2010). *Breaking the cycle: Effective punishment, rehabilitation and sentencing of offenders.* Cm 7972. London: HMSO.

Ministry of Justice. (2014). *Prisoners' childhood and family backgrounds: Results from the Surveying Prisoner Crime Reduction (SPCR) longitudinal cohort study of prisoners.* London: Ministry of Justice.

Morris, P. (1965). *Prisoners and their families.* London: George Allen.

Murray, J., & Farrington, D. P. (2005). Parental imprisonment: Effects on boys' antisocial behavior and delinquency through the life-course. *Journal of Child Psychology & Psychiatry & Allied Disciplines,* 46(12), 1269–1278.

Murray, J., & Farrington, D. P. (2008). The effects of parental imprisonment on children. In M. Tonry (Ed.), *Crime and justice: A review of research* (37, pp. 133–206). Chicago, IL: University of Chicago Press.

Murray, J., Farrington, D. P., Sekol, I., & Olsen, R. F. (2009). *Effects of parental imprisonment on child antisocial behaviour and mental health: A systematic review.* Oslo, Norway: Campbell Collaboration.

NNAPES. (2015). *The regional platform for the defense of the rights of children of incarcerated parents in Latin America and the Caribbean.* Retrieved from http://www.gurisesunidos.org.uy/presentacion-de-la-plataforma-nnapes-ante-la-audiencia-de-la-cidh

North Eastern Prison After Care Society (NEPACS). (1997). *The child and the prison: Proceedings of a conference held at grey college, Durham.* Durham: Author.

Peart, K., & Asquith, S. (1992). *Scottish prisoners and their families: The impact of imprisonment on family relationships.* Edinburgh: Scottish Forum on Prisons and Families.

Prison Population Statistics. (2017). Retrieved from https://www.gov.uk/government/statistics/prison-population-figures-2017

Quinton, D. (2004). *Supporting parents: Messages from research.* London: Jessica Kingsley Publishers.

Ramsden, S. (1998). *Working with children of prisoners: A resource for teachers.* London: Save the Children.

Richards, M. (1992). The separation of children and parents: Some issues and problems. In R. Shaw (Ed.), *Prisoners' children: What are the issues?* (pp. 3–12). London: Routledge.

San Francisco Partnership for Incarcerated Parents. (2015). *Children of incarcerated parents bill of rights.* San Francisco: San Francisco State.

Scottish Commissioner for Children and Young People (SCCYP). (2011). *Not seen. Not heard. Not guilty. The rights and status of the children of prisoners in Scotland. Review.* Edinburgh: Author.

Scottish Sentencing Council. (2017). *Children and the sentencing of parents: Report on discussion event with scottish sentencing council.* Edinburgh: Author.

Sedgman, K. (2017). *Influencing policy-making: How to engage governments with your research.* London: British Academy Newsletter. May 2017. Retrieved from http://www.britac.ac.uk/blog/influencing-policy-making-how-engage-governments-your-research

Seymour, C., & Hairston, C. (Eds.). (1998). Children with parents in prison. *Child Welfare: Journal of Policy, Practice and Program,* 77, 469–493. Special Issue.

Shaw, R. (1987). *Children of imprisoned fathers*. London: Hodder & Staughton.

Shaw, R. (1992). *Prisoners' children: What are the issues?* London: Routledge.

Shaw, S., & Crook, F. (1991). *Who's afraid of implementing Woolf?* London: Prison Reform Trust and The Howard League.

The Howard League. (2017). *Our legal cases*. Retrieved from http://howardleague.org/legal-work/our-legal-cases/

The Lammy Review. (2017). *An independent review into the treatment of, and outcomes for, Black, Asian and Minority Ethnic individuals in the Criminal Justice System)*: Gov.UK. Retrieved from https://www.gov.uk/government/uploads/system/uploads/attachment_data/file/643001/lammy-review-final-report.pdf

The Osborne Association. (2015). *See us, support us*. New York, NY: Osborne's Initiative for Children of Incarcerated Parents.

The White House. (2015). Retrieved from https://www.whitehouse.gov/blog/2015/07/15/president-obama-our-criminal-justice-system-isnt-as-smart-it-should-be

United Nations General Assembly. (1989). *The convention on the rights of the child*. New York, NY: Author.

Western & Pettit. (2010). *Collateral costs: Incarceration's effect on economic mobility*. Washington, DC: The Pew Charitable Trusts.

Index